D0314976

Smart Sitting

With Mindful Movement and Movement Maps

BRAIN TRAINING FOR SITTING
AND CONTROLLING BACK PAIN

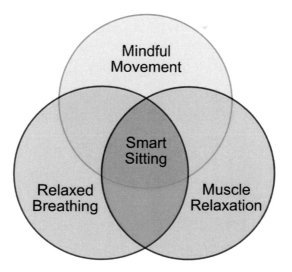

PETER DAVIES

About the Cover: Deep in thought and the back rigidly held in flexion, Rodin's Thinker illustrates the antithesis of smart sitting. The first large-scale bronze casting of The Thinker was presented to the public in 1904, a year after Dr Beevor presented his axiom in London when he concluded "only co-ordinated movements are represented in the excitable cortex".

Smart Sitting with Mindful Movement and Movement Maps
ISBN 978-1-909675-08-7
Published by Swan & Horn, Scotland 2017
Email: info@swanandhorn.co.uk

British Library Cataloguing in Publication Data: A catalogue record for this book is available from the British Library

Intellectual rights retained by the author
Smart Sitting with Mindful Movement and Movement Maps © Peter H. Davies 2017

All rights reserved. No part of this publication may be reproduced, stored in a retrieval system or transmitted in any form or by any means, electronic, mechanical, photocopying, recording or otherwise, without the prior written permission of the Publisher. For full details of our Archiving Policy, contact info@swanandhorn.co.uk.

Publisher's Disclaimer: Every effort has been made to ensure the accuracy of information contained in this publication, however no guarantee can be given that all errors and omissions have been excluded. The Publisher and Author accept no responsibility for loss occasioned to any person acting or refraining from action as a result of the content of this book. In following the techniques in the book, you assume all risk of injury to yourself, and release and discharge the Author from any and all claims or causes of action, known or unknown. You should not rely on this information as an alternative to medical advice from your doctor or other healthcare provider, or use this book if you have known serious or systemic pathology (generalised illness) or lower back pain as a consequence of a significant neurological deficit. If you have any specific questions about medical matters, you should consult your doctor or other health professionals before following the approach offered in this book.

Production, design and editing: Maria Hampshire-Carter assisted by Hannah Phillips.
Covers and graphic design: Peter H. Davies.
Printing and binding: Airdrie Print Services, Lanarkshire, Scotland.

Not for sale and not to be used in Canada, USA or Australia.

For my Mum, Daphne, who would say:
"Do your best, your very best,
and do it every day".

Praise for the book

"Peter is an exceptional Physiotherapist. I have been treated by him on and off for many conditions over the years. He is very open-minded and curious, with superb analytical skills, a very wide-ranging knowledge of healing approaches. His approach is steady and long-lasting, and he is committed in a humane but intelligent way to enabling patients to take control of their own healing process"— D. Micklem (Artist)

This comprehensive and well-researched book is illuminating and instructive for both professionals and patients. The author's experience and expertise is demonstrated on every page ... and his techniques will bring comfort to many— Lord Menzies (Ming) Campbell (The Right Honourable Lord Campbell of Pittenweem)

I could write page upon page about Peter's skills and knowledge as a clinician and his caring and pro-active personality. Yet I would still fall short of how his patient-centred, holistic and positive approach has given me a quality of life I was told was impossible – when all the other experts said "There is nothing else that can be done". He helps me keep focused using the tools described in Smart Sitting—L. Sutherland (Paramedic)

"I consulted Peter when I was suffering from lower back pain which was made a lot worse by the driver's seat of my new car. The concepts and exercises detailed in Smart Sitting were a brilliant help in relieving and managing my pain"—L. Semple (Podiatrist)

Reading this was like a light coming on. It clearly and simply explains and illustrates how back problems can be prevented or managed ... the guidance and recommended exercises in this book have allowed me to come off prescribed medication—M. Walker (Chairman of Walker Group Scotland)

Acknowledgements

Smart Sitting would not have been possible without those who encouraged me to persevere with the book and publish it.

I am especially thankful to William Ferguson, Mike Walker, Andrew Thompson and my eldest daughter, Lauren Davies, for their influential comments and advice during the early stages. Thanks, too, to the many unnamed people who have passed through my clinic and have helped me refine the practical application of these techniques.

I would also like to thank Alison Ireland, Georgina Lamrock, Damaris Micklem, Edmund Knox, Sarah Finlayson, Isobel Finlayson, Nicholas Phillipson, Sandra MacAskill, Kirsty Wheeler and Sylvia Wheeldon, who have provided valuable feedback on using the book; and to Maria Carter from Swan and Horn for her editorial and publishing expertise combined with her enthusiasm, support and conviction for making this book a reality. Big thanks are due to Linda Douglas for her patience and understanding when modelling for the photo sessions.

Above all, I want to thank my wife and best friend, Caroline Moffatt-Davies, who supported, challenged and encouraged me throughout the process, despite the amount of time this book has taken away from our family. And finally, I'd like to thank my youngest daughter, Sophie, burdened with disability, yet full of happiness and beautiful posture. You always surprise me.

Contents

1. Welcome to this book   1
2. How this book is different   3

PART ONE: KNOWLEDGE IS EMPOWERING

3. What you need to know about sitting   7
   Why sitting still is bad   7
   The perils of muscle tension   8
   Tension in your back and abdominal muscles   8
   Getting your breathing right   9
   Sensing your body's position   9
   Undesirable sitting habits   10
   The spine's centre position   10
   The present moment and brain training   11
   Delayed reactions and symptom flares   12
   Putting it all together   12

4. Your spine and how it moves (made simple)   13
   Bending forwards (flexion)   14
   Bending backwards (extension)   15

5. The role of movement maps   17
   Using visualisation to reduce pain   17
   Getting to grips with movement maps   18
   Mapping out your movements   20
   Mapping impaired movements   24

6. Problem sitting   27
   Pushing our limits in flexion   27
   What's wrong with "staying at the limit"   28
   What's wrong with "sitting up straight"   29

PART TWO: TIME TO RETRAIN

7. Learning to sit smartly – the learning process   33

8. The ideal sitting spine   35
   First, the ideal standing spine   35
   Now, the ideal sitting spine   36

9. Testing yourself before you start   37
   Feeling the effects of muscle tension   38
   Feeling tension when you sit   39
   Feeling how you breathe when lying   40
   Feeling how you breathe when sitting   41

Feeling how your pelvis moves when lying   42
Feeling how your pelvis moves on all fours   44
Feeling how your pelvis moves when sitting   46
Finding your "centre position"   47
Identifying habitual sitting positions   49

10. Mapping out your impairments   51
Mapping out your standing impairment   51
Mapping out your sitting impairment   53

11. Checking yourself to improve your competence   55
How feedback works   55
Moving the right parts   56
Giving yourself external feedback   57
Using internal feedback   60

12. Retraining your spine and your brain   65
Pitching yourself   65
The fundamentals   65
Exercise – duration and repetition   66
Using a softer surface   66
First things first – breathing and relaxing   67
Moving mindfully and comfortably   69
Simple pelvic rolling   70
Complex movements   73
Hours on a clock face   74
Letters of the alphabet   75
Flowing movements   76
Mixing it up   77
Working with your impairments   78

13. Taking your focus away from your back   81

14. Smart sitting in the real world   83
What is the ideal chair?   84
"Balanced" sitting in everyday chairs   86
Using a lumbar support   88
The position of the lumbar support   89
The angle of the seat-pan   90
The angle of the adjustable back-rest   91
Car seats and driving seats   93
Dealing with specific problems   94
Movement impairments   96

Closing comments   99
References and further reading   101
Index   107

1 Welcome to this book

This book has been designed as a concise, practical tool for people who want to have more awareness and control of their backs, particularly if they suffer from back pain, or want to improve their posture, increase their mobility and take the pain out of sitting.

The ideas and techniques presented here evolved from working with thousands of people suffering with chronic lower back pain. It is designed primarily as a self-help manual, but it can also be used in conjunction with a suitably trained therapist, and it provides a conceptual framework that will enhance your understanding of what, why and how to sit smartly.

This new smart approach applies to all kinds of sitting – in a chair, on a sofa, in the car, on a train or plane, or at your desk or at a meeting or conference – and will help you position and move your spine in a way that resembles what you do when you are standing or walking.

Ageing, and conditions like osteoarthritis and rheumatoid arthritis, are all associated with stiffness and pain, but if you have more back pain when you sit and less pain when you walk – like most of us do – then this book is very likely to be useful to you.

Often people in pain have a poor posture, little body awareness, a fear of movement, and low levels of activity. For them, sitting in one position for a long time tends to increase their pain, and they find that sitting habits prove a major barrier to the recovery and prevention of their back pain.

Creating meaningful and lasting changes in long-term postural habits doesn't happen with the help of a therapist alone – it's quite a journey for both the patient and the therapist, with the patient at the centre of that journey. My patients with back and neck pain quickly experience relief in their symptoms by using this approach and are easily able to change their sitting posture – often in as little as two weeks. Many have found significant improvements in their pain. In fact, for most (90% of people) with chronic back problems who feel better with gentle movement, rather than rest, this book will help.

How this book is different

The focus of this book differs from more conventional anatomical and physiological approaches that bombard you with details about anatomy and physiology, because it targets your movements and your awareness.[1] This is the mindful part. The fundamental aim is to increase your understanding of how you sit, and show you how to change your sitting habits. This will empower you to you achieve long-term benefits in your health and well-being.

The brain-training element involves restoring your awareness and control of your movements, enabling you to re-establish sensorimotor control of the neutral zone of your relevant "spinal segment". This might sound a bit technical at the moment, but it will all become clear.

A word of caution

I recommend that you read and understand this book before you try any of the tests or exercises. Above all, it is essential that any movements you try out are carried out without pain. If you start to feel pain during a movement, then change the size or direction of movement so you are moving within your comfortable range. This is not saying that pain is damaging the back, but moving *without* pain is more beneficial for training and recovery.

You should always begin trying out a new movement with fairly short sessions, of no more than two minutes at a time. If you make unfamiliar or uncontrolled movements repeatedly, you risk having a delayed reaction with increased pain and stiffness. In other words, there is a chance that your symptoms will get worse, so you must accept this risk before you undertake the movements outlined here.

Please do not rely on this information solely – consult your own doctor or other healthcare provider if you need to. If you know you have a serious or systemic illness, or lower back pain due to significant neurological deficit, then this approach may not be for you.

Again, you should seek advice from your doctor or a health professional before beginning.

PART ONE

Knowledge is empowering

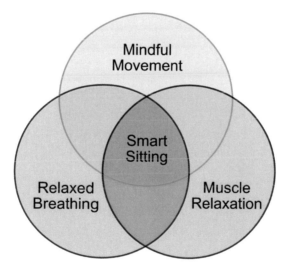

3 What you need to know about sitting

Sitting is *bad* for us – but it is pretty much unavoidable in modern life. Our bodies are designed for movement, and it has taken hundreds of thousands of years to evolve sufficient strength and mobility to function in a permanently upright position (unlike most mammals) which is quite a demanding stance!

Over the last few decades, our lifestyle of being on the move has given way to an inactive one[2] and this takes quite a toll on our spines. In fact, the average person now sits for more than five hours a day.[3] If we have to sit for so much of our time, we need to get smarter about it and become empowered to make an educated change to our day-to-day lives.

Sitting causes your pelvis to roll backwards and stops you from moving. Sitting still for a long time in a static posture – without moving – significantly contributes to back problems and muscle strain.[4]

Sitting may soon prove to be *the* major contributing factor to what is now a worldwide epidemic of chronic lower back pain. There is certainly a strong link between our less active lifestyles and the level of pain and disability we experience,[5] and it seems that prolonged sitting is also a clear risk factor for increased mortality – that is death from any cause.[6] An estimated 5.9% of all deaths could be attributed to daily total sitting time, even when physical activity is taken into account.[7] To be more precise, the estimated risk of all-cause mortality for sitting for ten hours a day is 52% higher than sitting for one hour a day. When moderate-to-vigorous physical activity is taken into account, the risk for sitting for ten hours a day is still 34% higher than sitting for one hour a day.[2,7]

Why sitting "still" is bad

Most of our daytime hours are spent sitting – to eat meals, to travel, to work and to relax, all of which promote inactivity. But there is a way to be more mobile through smart sitting. When modern ergonomics describe the ideal sitting position, they usually use diagrams that tend to reinforce the message of sitting in a fixed or static position – holding yourself with a rigid upright posture, usually with your hips and knees at 90°. Illustrations like this lead us to believe that an ideal sitting position should be maintained "statically", with little regard for movement or any awareness of our position in the seat.

The truth is that keeping still is neither sensible nor desirable. Not only does it deprive our bodies of the variability they need, but it also promotes stagnation to the circulation supplying the structural parts (building blocks) of the spine and increases unnecessary muscle tension.[8,9] What's more, when we become uncomfortable and find ourselves adjusting position from time to time, wiggling about on the chair, the movements of our lower back (lumbar spine) and our pelvis are usually poorly controlled[10] or are generally overlooked – or ignored altogether.

The perils of muscle tension

When you experience pain or injury, your brain and nervous system signal changes to your muscles to protect the affected part from further injury, and further pain.[11,12] This causes an increase in overall muscle tension, particularly in the large muscles of your trunk that serve to brace your spine.[13–16] While this may have some short-term benefits, they are outweighed by the potential for long-term problems, such as spinal compression, reduced mobility[17,18] and reduced blood flow to the structures and tissues in and around the back. Any prolonged, heightened tension in the muscles of your trunk can be very costly – both metabolically and mechanically speaking – and will probably exacerbate the pain in your lower back.[8,19–21]

Tension in your back and abdominal muscles

We are led to believe that we need a high level of muscle tension in our backs to control unwanted movements of our spine, but there is no conclusive evidence that this kind of stabilisation, often achieved by training or practising Pilates and other techniques, is superior to other forms of exercise for lower back pain.[22–26] It so happens that no studies carried out to date have demonstrated that lower back pain is due to instability of the spine. Despite a whole decade of active research, the concept of stabilisation of the spine is still only a theoretical model.[27]

What stabilisation training assumes is that you are able to choose which individual muscle can be activated in order to restrict and control your movements. The multifidus and transversus abdominis muscles have often been targeted with this type of training. However, the spinal cord and parts of our brain (namely, the cerebellum and the cerebral cortex) are not designed to contract isolated muscles.[28] Instead, the brain is primarily designed to control movement[29,30] – which is central to the approach used in this book, and highlights the need for mindful movements.

It is known that short-term increases in muscle activity for bracing the abdominal wall can be useful when you are bending or lifting a heavy object, for example, but not for the kind of low-intensity activity involved in sitting.[30,31] In fact, the opposite seems to be true – less muscular tension is known to be helpful when sitting when combined with good spinal alignment.[32] This means that as long as you sit with a relaxed, lengthened, well-aligned spine, and are able to move efficiently in that position, then your brain and neuromuscular system will work automatically to make whatever muscular adjustments are needed to achieve that position.[28,30]

Getting your breathing right

It is really important to breathe in a normal, relaxed way. Holding unnecessary tension in the muscles of your trunk and lower back increases the pressure in your abdomen and on your diaphragm (the sheet of muscle that separates your stomach from your lungs). This pressure disturbs the normal, relaxed breathing pattern, as do sensations of pain and anxiety.[33] When breathing becomes rapid and irregular, the level of carbon dioxide in the blood goes down, causing something called hypocapnia, which can lead to respiratory alkalosis.[33,34] This in turn can make your blood vessels constrict and reduce blood flow, especially to the heart and brain.[35] In this way, over-breathing can contribute to anxiety, fatigue, muscle pain and tightness – as well as problems with relaxing.[35] So, to prevent hypocapnia, you need to breathe in a relaxed and unconstrained way from your diaphragm – known as abdominal or belly breathing. This also helps you to relax, to reduce muscle tension and to reduce stress. You will be guided on breathing in Chapter 12.

Sensing your body position

Having awareness of the position of your body is known as "proprioception". Your brain can sense your overall position, as well as that of your head, limbs, hands and feet, and their movements, as well as your equilibrium (sense of balance). However, people who suffer from chronic pain in their lower back often end up with a poor awareness of the position of their lower back,[36] possibly because of changes in the organisation of the sensorimotor parts of the brain,[37–42] and this is despite the fact that people with lower back pain tend to think about their postures more than those who don't have it.[43]

You might be surprised to know that with chronic low back pain, the nerve cells in your brain that normally relate to your back can begin to extend into the areas representing your feet and legs![39] It is this "reorganisation" of your nervous system that causes problems with the movements you plan to make and the movements you actually make.[44,45] The result is pain.[46]

On top of this, if you have lower back pain, then your ability to reposition your spine is not very good,[36,47] which means you can end up always sitting in a bent-forward position (what we call flexed) without being aware of it. This also causes pain[14,47,48] and it increases the weight (or load) on your spine; and the more you bend the greater the load.[49] The good news is that awareness of movement and position can be improved with the right type of training.

Undesirable sitting habits

When you carry out activities you do all the time, like signing your name, driving a car, or walking, you don't have to think about them. They require little, if any, conscious thought and no awareness of the present moment to feel normal. These things are habitual for you, and the movements you make are automatic and subconscious – made in a default mode, or on autopilot. In the same way, you become unaware of the habitual aspects of your movements and posture – even if they are undesirable or lead to pain. The point is that it is much easier for your body to repeat habitual movements than to learn new ones. And this is where the challenge lies, because poor habitual sitting postures can trigger symptoms you would rather not have. Sitting in a stressful position without moving is one habit that tends to get seriously ignored, and it is one that needs to be identified before it can be tackled head on. The good news is that we can retrain our brains.

The spine's "centre position"

The spine is a strong structure that is most capable of withstanding loads when it is well aligned. This alignment is similar to the spinal curves seen when we walk or stand, with a feeling of gentle lengthening through the spine. Controlling and exercising in this position has the potential to prevent recurrent episodes of low back pain.[50]

This position is close to the so-called centred position of the spine, also called the neutral or mid position.[51] In this book, I use the term centre position, because it isn't a single dimension or passive position which the other terms suggest. It is a position that emphasises the potential for active movement in all directions – forwards and backwards, bending sideways, and rotation, or combinations of these.

Your spine has the greatest potential for movement from this centre position, unless disease, injury or the ageing process has put limitations on the range. The Alexander technique works at improving postural alignment and releasing unnecessary tension, aiming to improve function with less muscle tension,[52] which results in a reduction of pain symptoms. Musicians such as pianists often use this technique to obtain a good posture when sitting on a piano stool.

It is clear that our bodies are better at moving than staying still, but it is even better when our movements take place more often around the centre position. The approach used here involves actively exploring movements near the centre position, rather than focusing on static spinal alignment with muscle relaxation. The exploration of movement with good alignment rapidly improves the awareness and utilisation of the centre position.[53] However, the centre position varies from person to person, which means you will need to identify your own. The way to do this is described in Chapter 9.

The present moment and "brain training"

Most of the time, we plan future events or we recall things from the past – most of us give very little conscious thought to the present. The practice of mindfulness involves becoming more aware of the present.[54] It often encourages a focus on breathing because it is a simple and effective way to anchor attention to the moment. With practice, mindfulness is known to reduce the unpleasant sensations of pain and to reduce anxiety,[55] which in turn reduces pain.

Mindfulness can also be used for all kinds of physical activities, including movement. The mindful movement techniques outlined in this book are in fact "brain exercises". By building on your awareness of your body, they aim to improve both your conscious (aware) and your automatic (unaware) control of your lower back. Being "mindful" will allow you to track the tiny (pain free) moment-to-moment changes in position that create movement, so that you will be able to find comfortable positions while you are sitting, and they will become easier to find as you practise, and to use more often until they become habitual for you. This approach is a form of *brain-training* because learning new pain-free movement paths and patterns can create and reinforce new nerve pathways in your brain,[56] and restore the normal sensorimotor organisation of your brain. Nerves that fire together, wire together!

To train most effectively, you should begin with simple and achievable movements, usually around the centre position, and without pain[57] or unnecessary muscle tension. You will re-learn how to move in a relaxed and comfortable way – not to ignore or push through pain (the movements are not stretches). The old saying "no pain, no gain" has now given way to "know pain, know gain" and "no pain, no brain". In this way, you will begin to develop full and sustained awareness, and focus and concentration as you go through the various stages of learning.

Delayed reactions and symptom flares

As I mentioned previously, excessive repetitions of unfamiliar or poorly controlled movements can cause your symptoms to flare up even after you have finished doing the exercise. That is why you will be guided through a series of easy, short exercises lasting no more than two minutes, which you should initially carry out only two or three times a day. You will also be able to choose the right movements for you, with the emphasis on preventing flare-ups,[58] until you are able to repeat the movements more often and for longer without causing undesirable delayed reactions. Feeling stiff and sore after exercise does not indicate harm or damage to your body – it simply reflects the fact that your body is not used to the activity.[59] The role of feedback is very important in this process, which is covered in Chapter 11.

Putting it all together

When you retrain yourself and your brain to allow you to sit smartly, your controlled movements around the centre position will become automatic, relaxed, comfortable and pain-free. You will be able to relax and breathe from the diaphragm and sit with little effort. It will help you to have a basic understanding about movement and posture (covered in Chapter 4) and the stages of learning for new skills (Chapter 7).[60]

4   Your spine and how it moves (made simple)

The spine works in conjunction with your pelvis. The size and shape of the pelvis have a major influence on the position of your spine (lower back) when you sit. This is usually shown in complex anatomical illustrations, but I have used simple shapes here to describe how they work in a functional way, namely flexion and extension. This will give you a clear idea of the changes in position that occur during the testing and exercises which follow in Chapters 9 and 12.

The diagram below shows a simplified skeleton with the triangular pelvis meeting the base of the spine at the vertebra known as S1 (the topmost bone in the sacrum). This diagram also shows the pointed bones at the base of the pelvis known as the *sitting bones*.

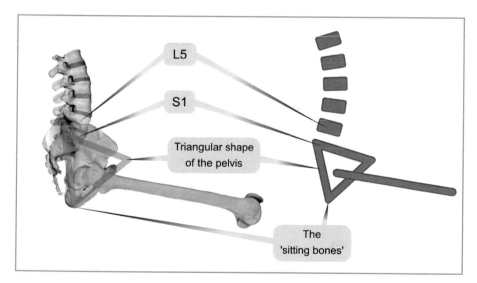

The S1 vertebra links to the lowest vertebra in the lumbar spine, known as L5. This is L5/S1, which is the target "target segment" for sitting used in this programme, and the one that the "centre position" relates to. Throughout the book, I simply refer to it as the *target segment*. It is circled in red in the diagram.

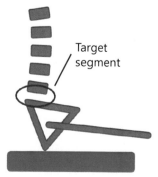

Bending forwards (flexion)

There is flexion of your lower spine, and the whole spine becomes C-shaped:

- When you stand and bend forwards.
- When you sit and bend forwards.
- When you roll your pelvis backwards.

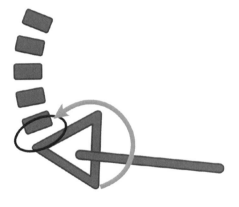

The C-shaped
curve of the spine.

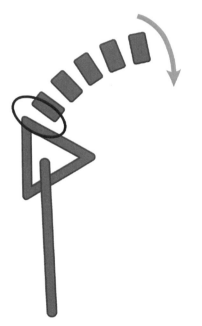

Standing and
bending forwards.

Sitting and rolling
your pelvis backwards.

Bending backwards (extension)

There is extension of your lower back, and the whole spine becomes a reverse C-shape (like a closing bracket):

- When you stand and bend backwards.
- When you sit and roll your pelvis forwards.

The reversed C-shaped curve of the spine.

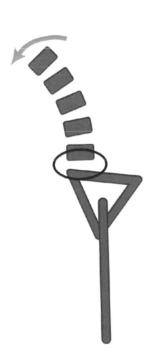

Standing and bending backwards.

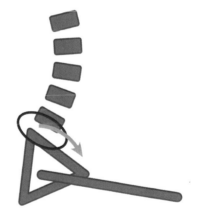

Sitting and rolling your pelvis forwards.

5 The role of movement maps

When there is acute or chronic back pain, certain movements cause pain, limiting how much we can move. Ageing generally reduces the range of possible movements, mostly the ability to bend backwards (extension). How much and what we can do also changes from day to day, depending on many factors, including the amount of pain experienced. However, when we know more about our own problems – our impairments – then we can identify the movements and positions that trigger our pain and other symptoms, and this contributes massively towards making long-lasting changes, both in our awareness of our movements and, very importantly, the way we sit. Smart Sitting is the result.

Using visualisation to reduce pain

Being able to visualise our movements makes moving more accurate and leads to a faster recovery from symptoms.[21,61] The problem is that, until now, it has been hard for people with back pain to form a mental image of the movements they make. The "movement maps" in this book will help you to form a picture of your movements, and highlight any areas of pain and movement impairments. This will help you visualise what is happening with your own back, as well as identifying the improvements you can make over time. The maps are especially useful for visualising your movements when you're sitting, and the position of the all-important target segment at the bottom of your spine (L5/S1), which is the lowest movable part of your back and one of the most common sources of pain. For people with movement impairments, regular training and awareness can improve their ability to move with fewer symptoms.

The basic map consists of four concentric circles as shown here. You can easily draw blank maps like these to map out different aspects of your back's movement. A few have been provided for you to use at the back of the book (page 110).

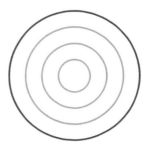

Getting to grips with movement maps

The four concentric circles on the map represent an "aerial view" of your range of movements at any one time, as if you are looking down at yourself in the centre. As in the diagram below, for all the maps shown on the following pages, imagine that you are standing in the middle and facing the top of the page.

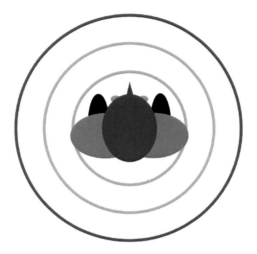

Standing upright in the centre circle represents no movement (or 0% of your possible range). The larger circles represent areas you can bend to or twist to from that position – they represent your *potential* movements in any direction. The further out (and larger) the circle, the larger the movement, thus the largest circle represents the *full extent* of your movement – but this is when you were a *young, mobile, healthy, symptom-free adult*. The extent of movement varies considerably from one person to another, because some people are just born to be more flexible than others.

The four circles (from the inside out) show *approximately* 25%, 50%, 75% and 100% of potential movement from your (0%) centre position. These percentages are just a rough guide for comparison when testing and monitoring yourself through the programme.

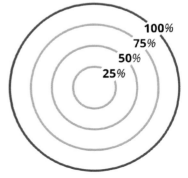

The uppermost parts of the circles relate to bending forwards (flexion) and the lower parts relate to bending backwards (extension) – as shown below.

The parts on the right side relate to leaning or twisting to your right, and the those on the left relate to leaning or twisting to your left. These are also known as "lateral" movements.

It's pretty simple.

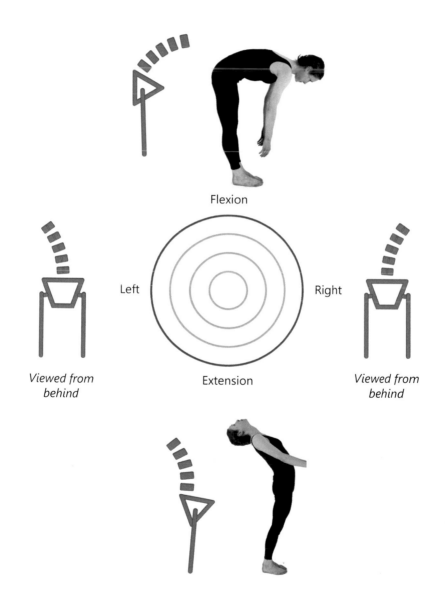

Flexion

Left

Right

Viewed from behind

Extension

Viewed from behind

Mapping out your movements

The movement maps can be used in a number of ways:

- To plan movements before you carry them out (future, planned and imagined movements).

- To track the position of the target segment while performing a movement (present movements).

- To plot out traces of movements you have carried out (past movements).

- To show where you have limited or painful movements (impairments).

- To help clarify why you have symptoms with some activities.

You can use them both to visualise your own movements, and add more details to highlight various aspects of those movements. Lines and arrows, for example, can be added to indicate the direction of future movements across your full range. The length of the line can be used to show the extent (range) of the movement.

Mapping "future" movements using lines and arrows

An arrow pointing to the top of the circles indicates that a forward bend (flexion) from the centre position is intended. This map shows full flexion (100%) of the spine from the centre position, achieved either by bending forwards while standing, or rolling your pelvis backwards when you are sitting.

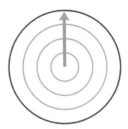

This two-headed arrow shows large movements made from the centre position, moving both fully forwards and fully backwards, through the centre position. In other words, 100% in both directions from the centre.

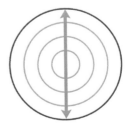

Here are small movements to each side, that remain close to the centre position (within 25%), thus reaching only the first circle.

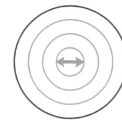

This is a series of movements starting from (and returning to) the centre position. In this case, they are tracing out the twelve numbers on a clock face, reaching 50% of the full range (the second circle).

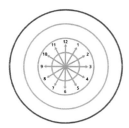

This map shows small side-to-side movements of the target segment in full flexion of approximately 100%. This is a common way to overload and injure your back. If the target segment is at, or remains near, an extreme of movement (in the outer circle), then other movements, such as side-to-side ones, will be limited.

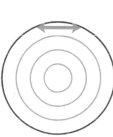

This map represents the complex movement involved in tracing the letter "a" in one smooth action.

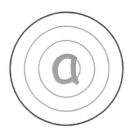

The position of the *target segment* at any one moment in time can be indicated on the map by a green dot.

Here the target segment (green dot) is in the centre position, in the middle of all four circles. This position has the greatest *potential* for movement in any direction, and is the strongest position for your lower spine to be in.

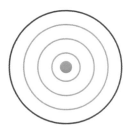

A green dot at the top of the map shows the position of the target segment in full flexion, such as when you stand and bend forwards to touch your toes, or when you sit and slump your spine into flexion (C-shape).

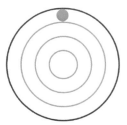

The dot on this map shows the position of the target segment during a forwards bend of somewhere between 25% and 50% of the possible range.

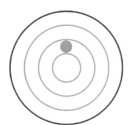

This map shows extension. Lying on your stomach can place the target segment in this position. This also happens when you lean backwards or tense your spine into extension (reverse C-shape).

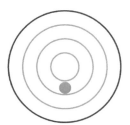

Past movements can be shown. Imagine the dot "burning" a path onto the map. This shaky line shows the path of the target segment and how the back was actually moving. It may follow an uneven path, jerking from side to side or at an uneven speed.

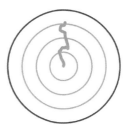

This squiggly line shows an area of many small variations in movement taking place when the spine is in a very flexed position. This can happen during sitting.

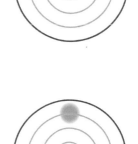

These changes in position over time can also be shown in the form of a green shaded area, as shown here.

This map shows the area of movements typically made when walking, in which the target segment is usually placed towards extension.

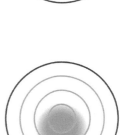

As explained previously, movement impairments occur when you move less than when you were a young, flexible, healthy, pain-free person. This may be because of ageing, pain, stiffness or fear avoidance (that is, a fear of feeling pain that makes you limit your movements). If your target segment moves into an area of impairment, or stays within an impairment (which is common when you sit), you are likely to increase your symptoms. After an "acute" injury to your back, the areas of impairment can change rapidly, resulting in reduced movement. This usually lessens as time passes, but some impairments are more resistant to change. Identifying your own type of impairment, and its extent, helps to explain your symptoms and allows you to make more comfortable movements.

The maps on this page show different kinds of impairments – their location (flexion, extension, or lateral) and their size (extent). They are indicated by the areas shaded in grey (the unshaded parts indicate areas that are *pain-free*). Once you identify your impairments on a movement map, you can add further information about any habitual movements and positions you use during specific activities, using dots and lines. This allows you to *predict* your own symptoms.

This map shows an impairment that mostly involves *flexion*. With these impairments, there are symptoms when you:

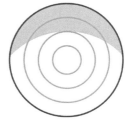

- Bend forward.

- Do activities like sitting to tie your shoe laces.

- Stay in a flexed position when sitting.

With *extension* impairments, as shown here, you will have symptoms when you:

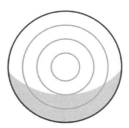

- Bend backwards.

- Do activities like walking, standing and swimming.

- Stay in an extended position such as lying on your stomach.

With *lateral* impairments (this map shows a right-sided impairment), your symptoms will occur when you bend or rotate to the right side by more than 50%.

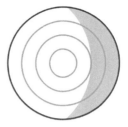

Multi-directional impairments can also occur. They tend to occur if you have an "acute" injury or problems associated with inflammation. Symptoms will occur whichever direction you bend or lean in.

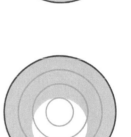

Combined impairments, as shown here, contain elements of all the impairments described above.

This is a large flexion impairment showing the position of the target segment (green dot) for someone staying still in a *flexed* position. It is common among people with chronic lower back pain when they sit, and usually increases their symptoms.

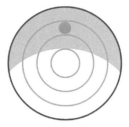

In the flexion impairment shown here, many small movements have taken place over time within the area of the impairment (green shading). Moving or staying still within this area is likely to worsen symptoms. Movements like this are discouraged when retraining.

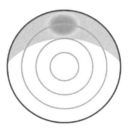

The shading on this map indicates many small movements made in extension (bending or leaning backwards). Extension often happens during standing, walking and swimming, and explains why people with flexion impairments are usually able to walk symptom free.

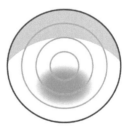

Even someone with a multi-directional impairment like this will be able to identify and move within (or stay still or exercise within) their unimpaired areas, which usually relieves symptoms. The arrows show an area of symptom-free movement that this person can aim for as they retrain.

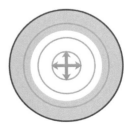

6 Problem sitting

This chapter outlines a few of the common sitting habits that most of us adopt in everyday life.

Pushing our limits in flexion

Most of us sit "habitually" with the target segment of our back held near its limit of flexion, as shown below. We tend not to notice that we are doing this until symptoms start.

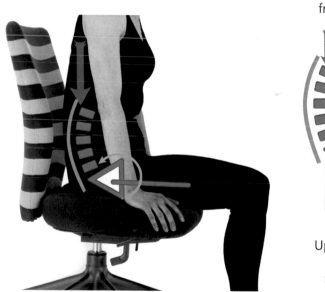

Downward pressure from the spine

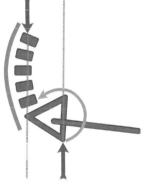

Upward pressure from the sitting bones.

Sitting usually results in a backwards roll of the pelvis and bending of the lower back into flexion (C-shape). The pelvis rolls backwards because there is downward pressure from the spine that falls behind the upward pressure from the sitting bones (orange arrows). The movement map representing this position is also shown.

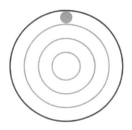

What's wrong with "staying at the limit"

When most people sit, their target segment and lower back stays near the limit of this fixed forward flexed position for a long time, with very little variation in movement, and with little awareness of their position.[48,62,63] This *lack of movement* and *lack of awareness of our position* is a major challenge for the lower back.

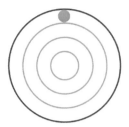

If you have a *flexion* impairment, as shown here, then sitting in this way will almost certainly increase your pain and other symptoms.

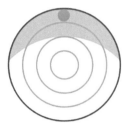

The same occurs if you have a *multi-directional* impairment.

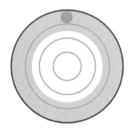

If you have an *extension* impairment, then sitting "habitually" in flexion will not increase your pain or symptoms.

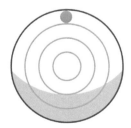

However, if your sitting habit places your spine in extension, then your symptoms will increase if you have an extension impairment.

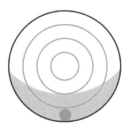

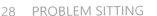

What's wrong with "sitting up straight"

When trying to maintain what we think of as a "good" sitting position, many of us unknowingly tense our muscles far too much. This results in a rigid and inefficient upright posture that quickly causes fatigue.

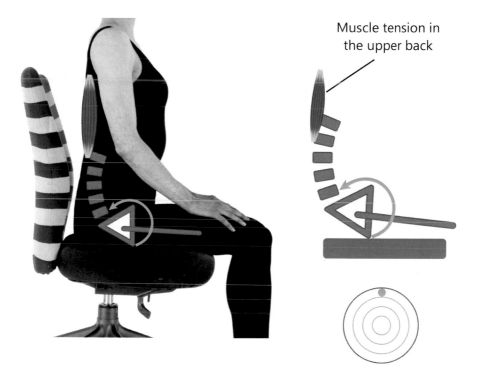

Muscle tension in the upper back

The increased tension in the back muscles, usually in the upper part of the spine, is shown by the red shading in the images above. The movement map shows that the target segment remains flexed.

Tensing the muscles in the upper back does little to correct the position of the flexed lower back, and actually reduces the movements of the upper back. It also has little influence on changing the position of the lower back.[64]

As well as this lack of movement, the increased tension in the upper back leads to stiffness, altered breathing and fatigue.

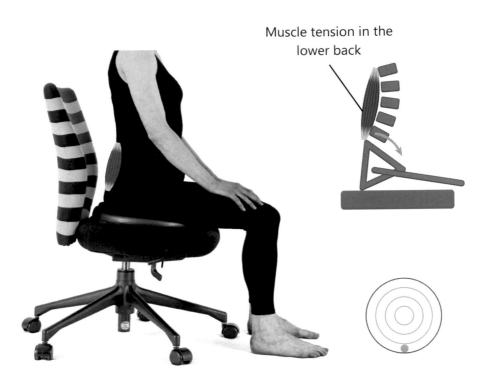

Muscle tension in the lower back

If the amount of tension is very strong in the lower back, as shown by the red shading above, it can hold your lower back *strongly* in extension – which reduces movement and increases spinal compression.

PART TWO

Time to Start Retraining

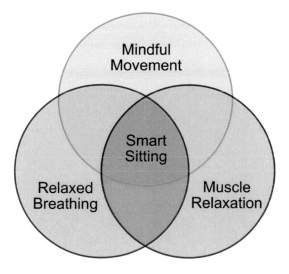

7 Learning to sit smartly — the learning process

There are four key "stages" of learning. You will go through each of them as you retrain yourself to sit smartly. In the first stage, you may be sitting in a slouched position all day without realising it. In the second, you will know that you are slouching, but not what to do about it. In the third, you will know how to sit better and that you need to practise – a lot. In the final stage, you will be sitting better (smarter) without having to think about it. The formal names for these stages are given below.

STAGE 1:
Unconscious incompetence

You are unaware that you don't know how to do something. This is covered in Chapter 9, in which you will **TEST** yourself to find out your ability to relax, breathe and move within your impairments.

STAGE 2:
Conscious incompetence

You become aware that you don't know how to do something – and it bothers you. It is covered in Chapter 10, in which you will be guided to **CHECK** whether you are doing things the *right* way.

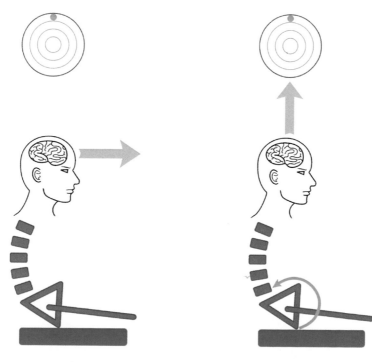

STAGE 3:
Conscious competence

During this stage, you are aware that you know how to do something, but it takes a conscious effort to do it. Chapter 11 shows you how can **RETRAIN** yourself accurately through focused awareness and mindful practice. You can now *choose* when and how to move and relax when sitting.

STAGE 4:
Unconscious competence

This final stage of learning marks the point when you are aware of how to do something and it becomes "second nature" to you. When you reach this level in this programme, you will be encouraged to **FOCUS** your active attention *away* from your back – for most of the time. Chapter 12 shows you how.

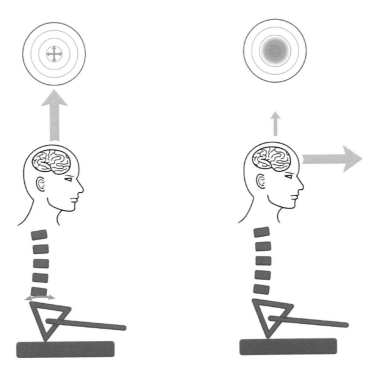

8   The ideal sitting spine

You usually have an ideal posture when you are standing or walking, when there is a relaxed lengthening throughout your spine from top to bottom, and your spine lies with a natural, gentle S-shaped curve. The top of the "S" is formed by the spine in the region just below the neck.

First, the ideal standing spine

When standing with this "relaxed lengthening", the alignment of the target segment should be spot-on. There is minimal tension in your muscles and maximum potential for movement.

If there is total relaxation of your back, you will slouch or stoop. However, if there is excess tension in your muscles, the spine will stiffen and reduce mobility. The point is that all of this happens without your conscious awareness.

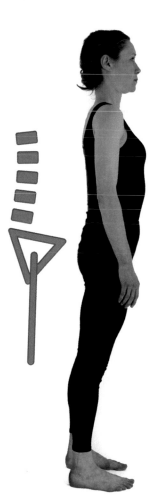

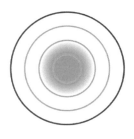

Now, the ideal sitting spine

When you sit, you want your spine to be as close as possible to the S-shape of standing. It is best if you:

- Don't hold your position rigidly, but aim for a relaxed upwards lengthening throughout your whole spine as shown below, using *just enough* muscle tension to maintain an upright position.

- Are able to make relaxed movements within the central area of movement, as shown by the green shading on the movement map, while maintaining good alignment of your spine.

- Breathe in a relaxed and unrestricted manner.

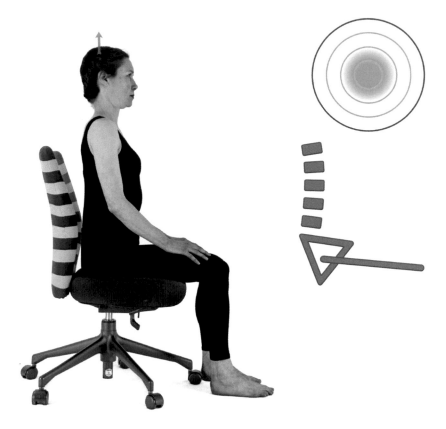

Ideally, there should be no discomfort or stiffness in your legs, and you should be able to move your upper back, as well as your hips and legs, in a comfortable and relaxed way that does not restrict your ability to position or move your pelvis.

9 Testing yourself before you start

Right now, you don't know how to start retraining yourself. The way for you to become *aware* of what you don't know is to carry out the following test movements. These simple procedures will help you identify which aspects of sitting are difficult for you.

Before you start, consider these questions:

- Do you really know what position your back is in when you are sitting?
- Do you know how often you move?
- When you move, can you move comfortably?
- Are your muscles tight?
- Do you have a good breathing pattern?

Then, when you have five minutes to yourself, choose a quiet, distraction-free place where you can sit or lie down comfortably. It is ideal to have:

- A large mirror positioned nearby so that you can see yourself making the movements as you sit.
- A clock or watch nearby, able to time 60 seconds.
- A chair with a soft surface or a thin cushion on it, or use a wobble cushion (page 66).
- A bed is useful for the lying-down exercises.

It will only take you a few minutes to go through all the tests in one go, and it is *extremely* useful to do this because it allows you to identify which issues are important for you and highlight which ones are more challenging. Then, when you start retraining, you can spend more time attending to the more troublesome ones.

In every test, you should avoid making any forceful movements – and make sure you keep them all comfortable and pain-free!

Feeling the effects of muscle tension

This is a simple way to appreciate how tension in your muscles can affect your movements.

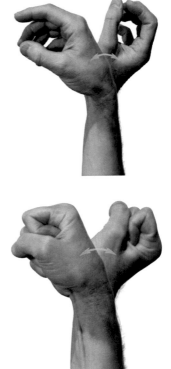

Hold one of your hands up in front of you and – keeping it relaxed – slowly move your wrist forwards and backwards. Focus on the feeling of movement *at the wrist*.

Now tighten your hand into a strong fist and move it forwards and backwards again. Was it easier to move your hand with your fist clenched or unclenched?

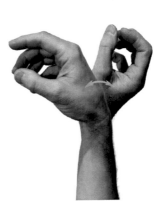

Now unclench your fist again and repeat the movements.

Did you notice the difference?

Try it again, this time with your eyes closed. And one more time, this time making fast and slow movements. This should make it clear that holding your muscles tensely makes movement more difficult.

Feeling tension when you sit

Sit comfortably towards the front of the chair seat, unless you are using one without a back support. Alternatively, sit on the edge of a bed.

Allow your muscles to "switch off" completely so that your back slumps a little.

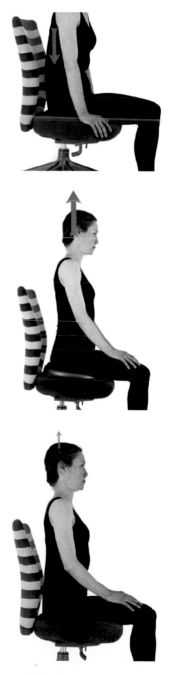

Now stretch your head and spine upwards, towards the ceiling (orange arrow) by tightening your back muscles firmly.

Can you feel how much effort you need to sit up straight?

Gradually reduce the amount of muscle effort while keeping the same curves in your spine and your head up. It can help to imagine a small helium balloon attached to the top of your head, lightly pulling your head and spine upwards. Now you should feel *relaxed lengthening* through your whole spine.

Feeling how you breathe when lying

Lie comfortably on your back on the floor or on a bed, with a clock that can time 60 seconds.

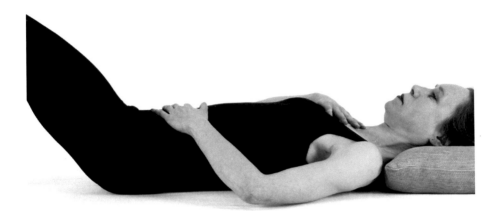

Place one hand over your abdomen and the other over your upper chest, as shown above. Now notice your breathing.

- When you take a breath in, notice where you breathe *first*. Which hand moves first – the one on your upper chest or the one on your abdomen?

- Then notice where you breathe *most*. Is there more movement in your abdomen, or your upper chest? Most of the movement should be in your abdomen.

- Now count the number of breaths you take in 60 seconds. The ideal is for 8 to 12 breaths per minute when you are at rest like this.

Feeling how you breathe when sitting

Sit up on the chair (with or without a back support) in a comfortable position, with a clock that can time 60 seconds.

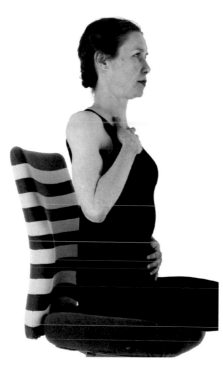

Place one of your hands on your abdomen and the other on your upper chest.

- Breathe normally and try to notice where your breathe in *first* from the movements of your hand – your upper chest or your abdomen?

- Notice where you breathe the *most* – is it through your upper chest or your abdomen? You should aim to breath through your abdomen.

- Count the number of breaths you take in 60 seconds. Between 8 and 12 breaths per minute is good.

Compare your normal way of sitting with *relaxed lengthening*, then when *slouching*. Do you feel a difference in your breathing? How does it feel compared with *lying down*?

Feeling how your pelvis moves when lying

Lie down on your back again, on the floor or on a bed, with your legs comfortably bent up. This position automatically places your lower spine close to the centre position.

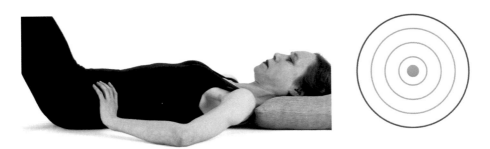

Place your hands on each side of your pelvis.

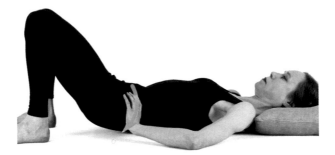

Gently roll (tip) your pelvis backwards, aiming for the C-shape of flexion, and feel your back moving towards the floor. This movement needs to be *large enough* for you to feel it, and *small enough* for you to stay comfortable. Stop the movement *before* you feel any discomfort.

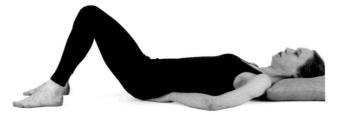

If you place both your hands under the small of your back and tighten your stomach to flatten your back towards the floor, you should feel the increased pressure on your hands.

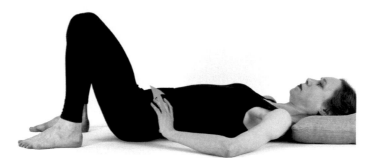

Gently roll your pelvis forwards again (into the reverse C of extension) and feel your back moving away from the floor. Again, this movement should be comfortable.

Now repeat this several times, gradually increasing the size of your movements in each direction to explore how far you can go while still free of pain.

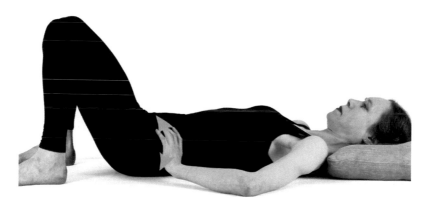

This movement map shows the type of movements you are aiming for during this test – just small movements that don't challenge you, or feel forceful, or reach into the areas of your impairment.

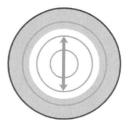

Looking at a mirror to see your back may make it easier to do the movement.

Feeling how your pelvis moves on all fours

A flat, stable, comfortable surface is best for this test. You can place a folded towel under your knees or move onto a soft carpet or rug. A firm bed is also suitable. If your wrists are sore when the palms of your hands are in contact with the floor, use either hold a rolled-up towel under your palms or make a fist with each hand and rest on your knuckles.

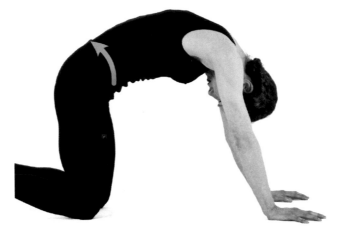

Gently roll your pelvis backwards into flexion (C-shape) so that your back moves away from the floor. Only do this slightly to begin with, so that you stay within your *comfortable* range. Try to minimise the movements of your shoulders, neck and upper back.

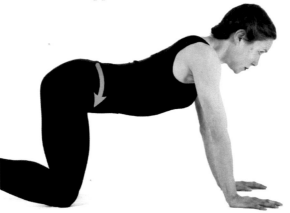

Now gently roll your pelvis forwards into extension (reversed C-shape), so that your back moves towards the floor. Your stomach should be relaxed so that it sags downwards. Again, try to move your shoulders, neck and upper back as little as possible.

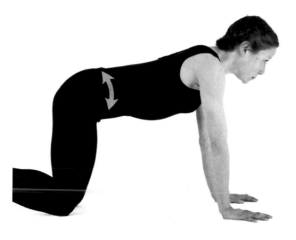

Repeat this several times in both directions, gradually increasing the size of movements to explore the amount of movement that is free of pain.

This movement map shows you the kind of movements you are aiming for; they shouldn't extend into the region of your impairment.

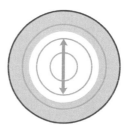

Feeling how your pelvis moves when sitting

Now sit back on the chair, in an upright position with a feeling of relaxed lengthening of your spine.

Place your hands comfortably on your thighs and, using *small* movements, roll your pelvis forwards, then backwards, as shown on the inset movement map.

Try to minimise the forwards and backwards movements of your head and shoulders.

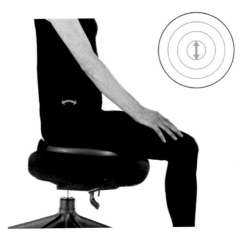

Gradually increase the size of your movements to explore your range of comfortable movement, as shown on the map. If you place your hands on your hips, you will feel the rolling action more easily.

Notice how much movement you can make in each direction, *without pain*. You may find that one direction is more comfortable than the other.

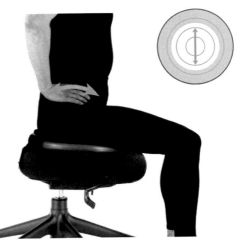

If you cannot easily feel these movements, you could try sitting on a softer surface, or you could try a wobble cushion (page 66).

Looking in a mirror to see your back may make it easier to do the movement. Other forms of external feedback can also be used (page 57).

Finding your "centre position"

This is the *most important* position to identify when sitting, as retraining is based on the movements that take place relative to the centre position. Because there is a natural tendency for your spine to drift into flexion when sitting, you will often need to check your centre position.

Stand comfortably upright with the chair behind you, and the mirror to one side of you so that you can see the curves of your back.

Aim to feel a relaxed lengthening through the whole of your back. This is the "centre position" which produces a natural, gentle S-shape of your spine. You should not slouch or hold yourself rigidly with excess muscle tension. Your breathing should be relaxed and easy.

Now spread your fingers of both hands and place one on your abdomen. Place the other over the small of your back. This will allow you to monitor the position of your lower back.

The mirror will help you compare and monitor the position of your spine as you change position.

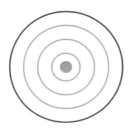

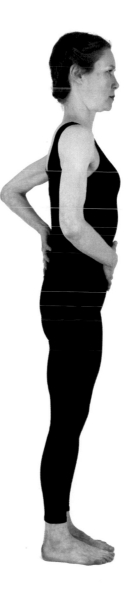

Gently lower yourself down into a sitting position on the chair, while keeping your hands in place, and maintaining the relaxed lengthening of your spine.

Monitor the position of your back and the movement that takes place as you sit down.

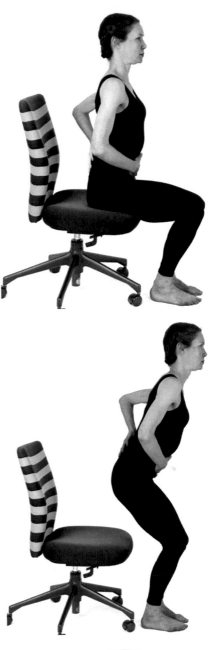

Then gently stand up again.

Repeat this five more times, all the time noticing any changes in the position of your back with your hands.

This movement map shows how the centre position is maintained throughout this move.

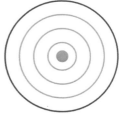

Identifying habitual sitting positions

Sit in your "usual" way in a chair or on a sofa that you use often. Sit for a few minutes until it feels "normal" for you. This is your starting (habitual) position, the details of which are currently unknown to you.

Try to notice how your starting position compares to the centre position (page 47).

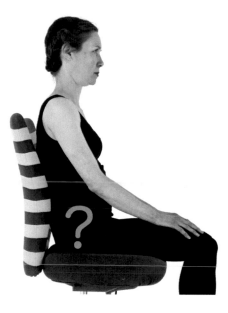

Without causing symptoms or discomfort, slowly roll your pelvis backwards then forwards from your starting "habitual – through the centre position.

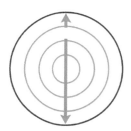

Now *estimate* how much movement was available in each direction from your starting position and mark it on a movement map with an arrow. You can also check your sideways (lateral) movements by rolling the top of your pelvis to the left and right.

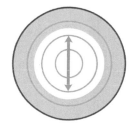

This movement map shows someone with a habitual position that is in flexion, which allows a lot of forward rolling of the pelvis into extension, but very little backward rolling into more flexion.

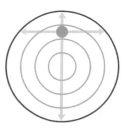

10 Mapping out your impairments

This is where you find out how much comfortable movement you have when standing or sitting. We start with standing because it is easier to see and test your movements when the movement takes place above the target segment (L5/S1). When testing yourself when sitting, the movement is from the pelvis and takes place below the target segment. For this reason, your standing map and sitting map may look different. Your impairments can also be mapped out in other positions – lying down, in a bed, or when leaning on "all fours". The two main tests are described here. Additional movement maps are provided on page 110.

Mapping out your standing impairment

Stand upright, in the centre position with relaxed lengthening and relaxed breathing.

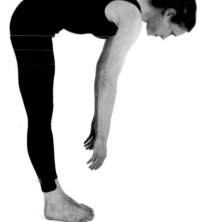

Gently bend forwards towards your toes (into flexion). Stop moving at the *first* sign of pain or stiffness. Then slowly return to a standing position.

Estimate *roughly* how far you were able to move compared to what you would expect if you had no pain or stiffness. Remember that the circles represent 25%, 50%, 75% and 100% of your potential range.

Mark this with a dash on the blank movement map on page 54. Thus your map should represent "as far as you can move comfortably" before you reach an impairment.

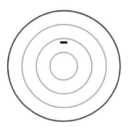

Range of movement is very individual and should not be compared with that of other people. The map shown here represents a forward-bending limit of about 50%.

Now stand upright, with your spine in the centre position, and lean backwards – gently and *comfortably*. Stop at the *first* sensation of pain or stiffness.

Stand fully upright again and mark a dash for this movement on your own movement map (page 54).

Then lean comfortably to your left and back to the centre, and add another dash.

Then lean to your right and back to the centre, and mark it.

You should now have four dashes on your map, as shown in the example below.

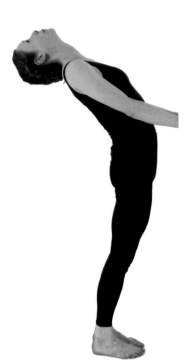

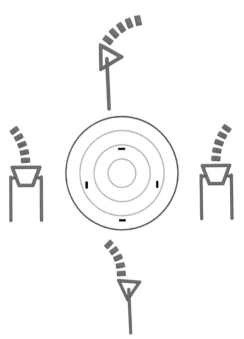

When you have all four marks on your movement map, join them together and shade the area that falls *outside* the marks, all the way to the edge of the largest circle, as shown in this example. This represents your *standing impairment*.

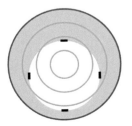

Mapping out your sitting impairment

Sit back on the chair (with or without a back support) in a comfortable upright position, with a feeling of relaxed lengthening of your spine.

Gently roll your pelvis backwards into flexion (C-shape), and stop at the first sensation of pain or stiffness. Then return to the starting position. Mark your estimated extent of movement on the second blank map on page 54.

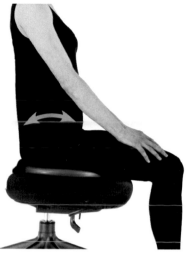

Now *gently* roll your pelvis forwards into extension (reverse C-shape), estimate your extent of movement and return back to the centre, and mark a dash on the map.

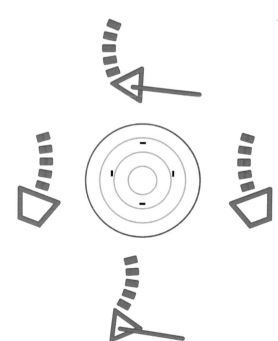

From the starting central position, tip the top of your pelvis to your left, and back to the centre, and add another dash on the *right* side of the movement map (as the left side of your body lengthens and the right side shortens the target segment moves to the right).

Then tip the top of your pelvis to the right, and add another dash on the *left* side of the map.

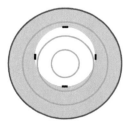

You can then join all four marks together and shade the area *outside* them. This represents your *sitting impairment*.

Your standing impairment

Add the four marks to the circles then shade the area that lies outside them. This movement map represents your standing impairment.

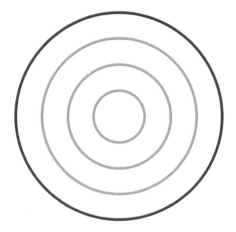

Your sitting impairment

Add the four marks to the circles then shade the area that lies outside them. This movement map represents your sitting impairment.

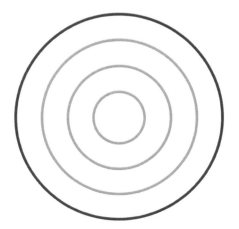

11 Checking yourself to improve your competence

In this part of the learning process you will check the movements you tried out in Chapter 9 until you to know how to do them *easily*. You are probably not sure whether you've really got the hang of them yet, but by aiming for "conscious incompetence" you will progress quickly. The fastest way to get there is by getting *good feedback*.

How feedback works

Good feedback allows you to monitor the accuracy of your movements while you are retraining.[65] You begin with *external* feedback – that is, external to the *internal* feedback from the sensations in your back or spine. Options include:

- Placing your hands over the part you are moving.
- Using mirrors to watch yourself.
- Recording yourself with a mobile or video camera.
- Getting direct guidance from a trained therapist.

Getting feedback *during* your movements is especially valuable because seeing your back in motion results in less lower back pain and rapid resolution of symptoms.[61] However, in the long term, relying on *external* sources of feedback like this is not practical, nor is it desirable if you want to become fully independent.

As you continue retraining, it is important to shift away from external feedback to *internal* feedback, which involves tuning your brain into the sensations and signals from the structures within your back, thus allowing it to process those signals. Gaining more awareness of your body in this way will make it easier for you to sense the position of different parts of your body relative to each other.

Restoring this awareness of movement comes from accurate training, with movements that we are able to notice on a moment-by-moment basis. And with improved body awareness, we become more aware of our position and movements, activating both the conscious and automatic pathways that are needed for the activities and tasks of everyday life. This is why it is so important to make *mindful* movements for a while.

Moving the right parts

Your movements should occur from your pelvis, which is essential for controlling the target segment for sitting. As you move your pelvis in any direction, try to minimise any forwards or backwards movements of your upper back (thoracic and cervical spine) and your head and shoulders. You should also not let your legs or feet move too much.

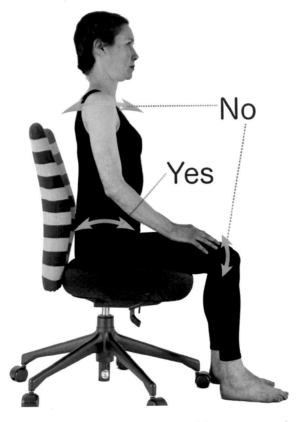

If you watch yourself and find you are making unwanted movements, it may be because:

- You have high muscle tension in your lower back, causing your back to be more rigid (try changing your position so you are better able to relax, or try lying on your back with your legs bent).

- You are breathing in a way that is not relaxed (check your breathing pattern and spend some time practising it before trying to move).

- You have very tense abdominal muscles (try doing more relaxation).

- Your attention is focused elsewhere (don't worry about it — just gently return your thoughts to the present moment and focus your attention on the area you want to move).

- You are simply not used to moving your lower back (you will have to practise the movement or try moving in a different position).

Giving yourself external feedback

With your hands on your sides

Sitting safely and comfortably on a chair with a soft surface *without* a backrest, place your hands on each side of your pelvis, with your fingers pointing forwards, towards your stomach, and your thumbs curving towards your back. (See page 66 to find out more about sitting on a soft surface.)

Roll your pelvis backwards (into flexion). As you roll, feel your fingers move up and your thumbs move down. Return to the centre position.

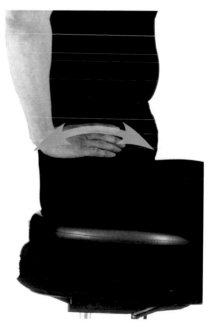

Then roll your pelvis forwards (into extension) so that your fingers move down and your thumbs move up. Return to the centre.

Tilt your pelvis to one side, and back to the centre, and then to the other side. Notice how one hand moves up while the other moves down.

Keep checking your movements in the mirror to make sure there is minimal sideways movement of your upper back, head and chest.

You can also do this lying down, with your hands in the same positions.

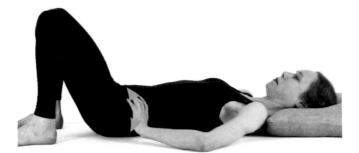

With your hands on your front and back

Sit comfortably on a chair *without* a backrest. Put the palm of one hand on your abdomen and the other on the small of your back, with your fingers spread out wide.

Roll your pelvis backwards (into flexion) and, as you roll, feel both your hands move backwards. The fingers of the hand on your back may spread apart even more. Return to the centre position.

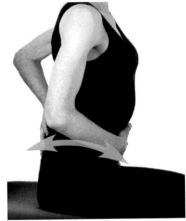

Then roll your pelvis forwards (into extension) and feel your hands move forward. The fingers over your abdomen may spread out further. Return to the centre position.

Try this too when you are lying down, with both legs comfortably bent, and both hands under the small of your back. As you roll your pelvis backwards (into flexion) you will feel more pressure on your hands. Rolling it forwards will lessen the pressure on your hands as your back extends.

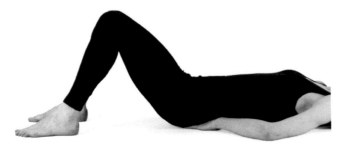

With visual aids

Use a mirror or a live video feed to get immediate feedback on your movements and the position of your lower back. This also lets you compare the curve in your lower back when you are standing and when sitting. Watching the rolling movements of your pelvis means you can check for unwanted movements of your head, arms, chest, legs and neck. Photographs and video footage can also be useful for revealing large differences between what feels "normal" and the actual position of your lower back. A "close-up" of your back when you sit often reveals that there is far more flexion than you might expect.

With pointing devices

This method of visual tracking is good for showing the fluidity and smoothness of your movements, as well as their speed and extent. A torch with a tightly focused beam can be attached to a belt around your waist, at the top of your pelvis. Point the torch forward, so that when you face a wall, it makes a spot that moves as you move.

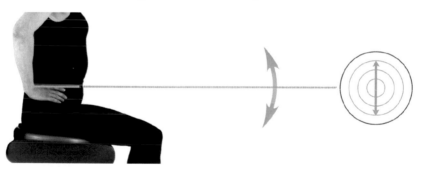

It will move upwards as you roll your pelvis backwards (into flexion). It will move downwards as you roll your pelvis forwards (into extension).

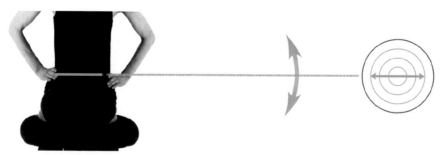

If you move the torch so that it is pointing to the side, it will trace out the sideways movements of your pelvis.

Working with a therapist who is trained in techniques like the ones shown here can help you learn new skills quickly.[55] By careful placement of their hands, therapists are able to guide your movements and help you *feel* them more easily. They also have experience in giving instructions, using imagery, and other little tricks like applying adhesive tape to your lower back so that it pulls on the skin when you bend.

Do remember, however, that therapists *cannot experience* what you are feeling physically, so ultimately you have to rely on your own internal feedback to perfect your movements.

Giving yourself internal feedback

Mentally rehearsing a movement before you actually carry it out will help you improve the quality of that movement. It also improves your level of awareness and your ability to feel the movements you make.

Imagine a bowl of water

Imagine that your pelvis is a bowl filled with water. When you are in the centre position, the water stays level in the bowl. When you roll your pelvis back (into flexion), the water spills over the back edge. When you roll your pelvis forwards (into extension), the water spills over the front edge.

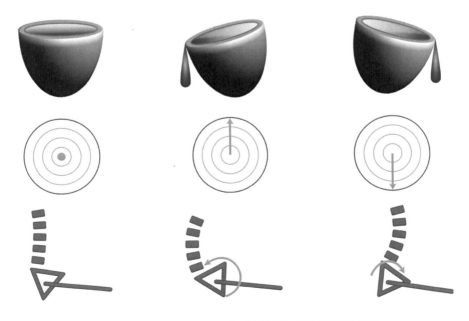

Imagine a pencil

Imagine a pencil is attached to the top of your pelvis (at the level of the target segment) and pointing down to the floor as you sit in the centre position.

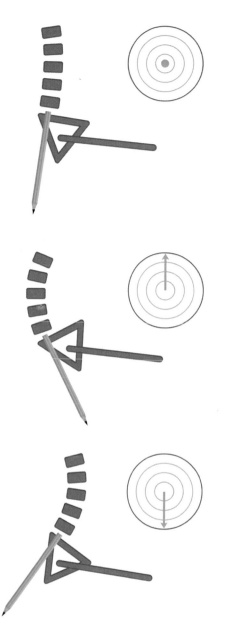

When you roll your pelvis backwards (into flexion), it will trace a line from that point towards the front.

When you roll your pelvis forwards (into extension), it will trace a line from that point towards the back.

Imaginary lines drawn by the imaginary pencil can be marked onto a movement map.

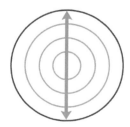

You can also change the orientation and site of this imaginary pencil to make the exercises more or less difficult for you. Thinking of movement from the top of the pelvis tends to be easier.

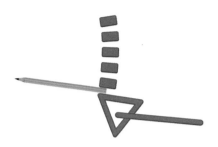 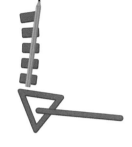

Imagine a pivot point

Focus your mind on the *point of contact* that is made when you sit upright on a chair, that is your sitting bones at the bottom points of your pelvis.

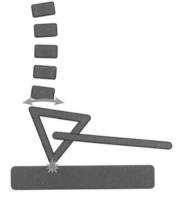

Now imagine that those points form a *fixed pivot* for moving your pelvis, shown here by the orange star.

Imagine this pivot point as you roll the top part of your pelvis forwards and backwards.

Imagine a movement map

Imagining the movement of the green dot on a movement map can help you picture the moment-to-moment changes in your position.

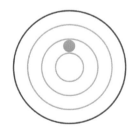

You might picture this dot as it traces out a number "8" or you might focus on the speed and direction of the dot as it moves through any movement path. It can be helpful to imagine a specific movement path on the map, and think "how do I get it to move like that?".

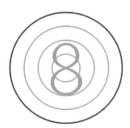

You can also compare the accuracy of your planned movement paths with how the movement was performed.

Did the movement occur in the right direction, at the right speed and the right range of movement?

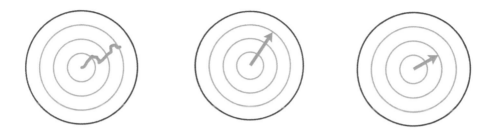

Close your eyes

When you practice movements with your eyes closed, you will shield yourself from outside distractions and help your mind to focus on what you are feeling and what you are doing.

12 Retraining your spine and your brain

Now you are well on the way to "conscious competence". You are aware how to do the movements, but they still take some effort. From this point on, you will need to practise with accuracy and repetition, using mindful movements. You will focus on one issue at a time, preferably starting with the more difficult ones that you identified in Chapter 9.

Pitching yourself

Your training sessions should not be *too easy* or involve automatic or habitual movements – they will not help you learn or develop the new skills you need. And if they are *too difficult*, you will become frustrated or do them inaccurately.

Simply aim to train at a level that is comfortable, yet still challenging. You will be able to step up the level of challenge when you want to.

The fundamentals

Before starting to train, you must be able to breathe well, whether lying or sitting. The importance of relaxed breathing *should not* be underestimated, and you should avoid holding your breath at all times.

You must also be easily able to relax and allow your spine to gently lengthen in a relaxed manner. Bear the following points in mind as you go through the exercises.

- Make sure you choose a safe flat surface that provides comfort and support for all the positions.
- Reduce any unnecessary muscle activity *anywhere* in your body.
- Aim for a relaxed lengthening throughout your spine as you find the centre position.
- Consider the area of movement you want to retrain (usually around the centre position).

If moving near the centre is a problem for you, then target the training area *slightly away* from the problem – usually in the direction opposite your impairment. For example, you may need to work more towards flexion if you have a major extension impairment, or work more towards extension if you have a major flexion impairment (page 96 and 97).

- Focus on comfortable, pain-free movements of your pelvis – not your lower back.
- Use feedback to check you are moving accurately.

Exercise duration and repetition

Try to do these training exercise "little and often". When you are starting out, only practise for two minutes at a time, but do this two or three times throughout the day.

Make sure that you are *kind* to yourself. If you cannot get something to work, leave it for a bit, then try again later. When you practise and become more familiar with the movement, there is less chance of triggering a delayed reaction (page 3 and 12), which means you will be able to repeat the movement more often and for longer.

Using a softer surface

You can use a soft cushion, a "wobble" cushion or an empty water-bottle with some air in it to carry out the sitting movements. These aids can be especially helpful for side-to-side movements because the unstable surface they provide allows you to feel the movements more easily.

As your training progresses, they will no longer be needed, and you can use your new skills on *any* sitting surface.

Note that special care is required to keep your balance on very soft surfaces like these, to prevent you from making uncontrolled movements that can provoke your symptoms.

- You can place your hands on the seat or armrests to steady yourself.
- Don't fall off the chair!

First things first – breathing and relaxing

Breathe from your diaphragm in a relaxed and unconstrained way – with abdominal (*belly*) breathing. As you breathe in, the diaphragm flattens to bring air into the base of your lungs, and the abdomen expands and rises. As you breathe out, the diaphragm relaxes and curves into the chest, allowing the abdomen to lower and the air to leave your lungs.

Relaxed breathing while lying

Lie on your back in a comfortable position, using pillows for support under your head and knees if required, and place your hands on your abdomen. Close your eyes if it helps.

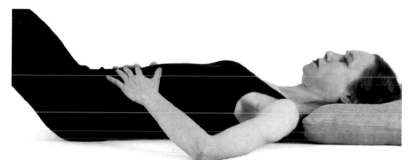

Breathe gently through your nose (if you can). Each breath should be smooth and even on both the in-breath and the out-breath. Your mind may drift onto other thoughts; simply notice how it chases new thoughts and *gently* return your attention to your breath. Do not increase the depth of your breathing. Feel your abdomen slowly rise and fall, and keep noticing the *rhythm* of your breathing. You may need to occasionally check the rate and location of your breathing (page 40).

As you progress:

- Focus your mind on relaxing the areas of your body that are holding tension.

- Keep your breath smooth and even and aim for a relaxed pattern of 3 seconds in and 3 seconds out.

- Try breathing in for 3 seconds and out for 7. This should help you to relax even more.[66]

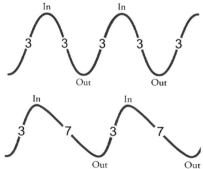

Sit on a chair, with or without a backrest, with relaxed lengthening of your spine and your pelvis close to the centre position. Place both hands across your abdomen. They can be removed later.

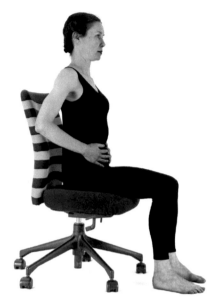

Breathe gently through your nose, and feel your abdomen slowly expand and relax, while noticing the rhythm of your breathing. Do not increase the *depth* of your breathing.

You may need to occasionally check the rate and location of your breathing (page 41).

As you progress:

- Focus on relaxing the areas of your body that are holding tension – including your stomach and abdomen.

- Keep your breath smooth and even and aim for a relaxed pattern of 3 seconds in and 3 seconds out.

- Try breathing in for 3 seconds and out for 7. This should help you to relax even more.[66]

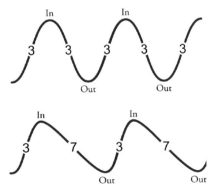

Moving mindfully and comfortably

To avoid being distracted, train in a quiet, comfortable, warm environment, closing your eyes from time to time. The key to moving mindfully is to think "How do I get my pelvis to move like that?" and to use some sort of mental imagery to visualise the movements you make. For example you could imagine a green dot moving across a movement map, to show the smoothness, speed, direction and extent of the movement. Visualising like this focuses your mind and lets you follow your movements on a moment-by-moment basis.

As you progress

When you're able to complete a particular movement in a controlled and easy manner, you can increase the level of difficulty in several ways.

- Try other positions. Improving in one position allows your body and brain to apply the new skill to other positions and contexts.

- Train for longer times and more frequently.

- Make more subtle movements. These are more difficult to feel, so close your eyes to help. As you improve, the movements will become smoother and flow better. Carry out complex, smaller, slower, more relaxed and controlled movements both when sitting or standing, and monitor them using internal feedback, and keep checking you are moving accurately.

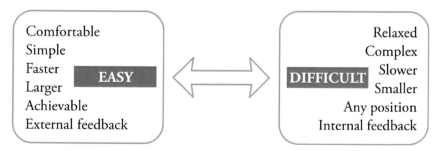

Comfortable			Relaxed
Simple			Complex
Faster	EASY	DIFFICULT	Slower
Larger			Smaller
Achievable			Any position
External feedback			Internal feedback

Try not to rush through these exercises. It is important to take your time and pay attention to their *quality*. After several weeks of working in an area that is comfortable and *pain free*, the impairment usually recedes as you improve. However, some chronic impairments are more resistant to change than others. These often benefit from controlled "graded" stretching (page 78) into the impairment. Do not be tempted to start stretching into the impairment before you have good and habitual control of movement around the centre position.

Simple pelvic rolling

When lying down

Lie on your back on the floor or your bed with your legs comfortably bent by drawing your feet towards you. Place your hands over each side of your pelvis to make it easier to feel your movements. Alternatively, place one hand beneath the small of your back (page 42). As you tighten your stomach to flatten your back towards the floor (or bed), the pressure on your hand will increase. Make sure you stay comfortable before you start to move.

Roll your pelvis backwards (into flexion) and feel your back move towards the floor or bed.

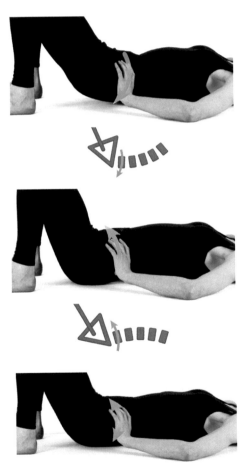

Roll your pelvis forwards (into extension) and feel your back move a way from the floor or bed.

Continue doing this in both directions for about two minutes. Focus on the amount of movement you are able to make without feeling any dis-comfort. This helps reduce fear avoidance and starts the process of movement awareness.

Remember to control the size of your movements to minimise any discomfort. They should be comfortable and inside your area of impairment.

When on all fours

With this movement, you should try to minimise the movement of your shoulders, neck and upper back. Rest on all fours on a comfortable, stable surface and close your eyes.

Roll your pelvis backwards (into flexion) without discomfort, and feel your back moving away from the floor. This small arching of the back is like a cat stretching.

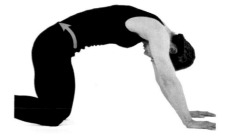

Roll your pelvis forwards (into extension) and feel your back and stomach move towards the floor. Your stomach should be relaxed and allowed to sag.

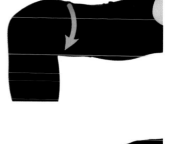

Start with small movements and gradually increase them to explore your range of comfortable movement.

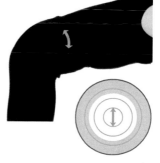

Continue for about two minutes and make sure that your breathing and back muscles also feel relaxed.

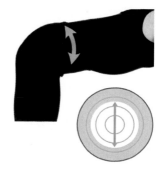

When sitting

These movements are easier to feel when sitting on a very soft surface or a wobble cushion (see the note and word of caution on page 66 about sitting on a soft surface). If the chair has a backrest, do not lean back against it. This can be done at a later stage of training. For now, just focus on the size of your movements and feel the extent of pain-free movement that you have. Sit comfortably upright on the chair with relaxed lengthening of your spine.

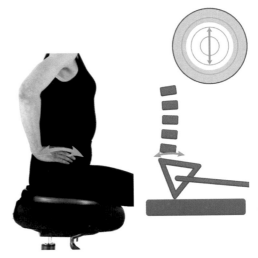

Roll your pelvis forwards and backwards without discomfort.

Explore this movement for about two minutes.

Your movements should be comfortable and inside your area of impairment.

As you progress

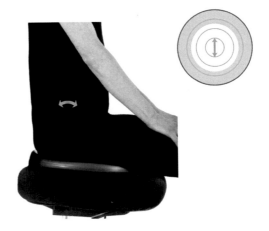

- Try to make your movements smooth, fluid and relaxed.

- Slow down your movements and notice what happens to the tension in the surrounding muscles.

- Roll your pelvis forwards and backwards over a smaller range, until the movements are just small enough for you to still be aware of them.

Complex movements

Complex movements are easier to do if you think about movement from the top of the pelvis – here an imaginary pencil would be pointing upwards (rather than downwards for a normally orientated Movement Map) and produce an incorrect movement map. With these movements, it is more important to explore and enjoy comfortable, relaxed movement.

Points on a compass (North South East West)

Sit comfortably on a chair with or without a backrest, with your hands on the top of your hips.

Slowly and gently roll the top of your pelvis to the left. As your right buttock lifts away from the seat, the right side of your pelvis will move up towards your right shoulder. You may notice that your pelvis tilts and shifts towards the left.

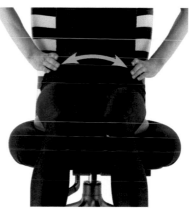

Return to the centre position and repeat to the right. Return to the centre position and roll the top of the pelvis backwards, then return to the centre position and roll the top of the pelvis forwards.

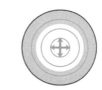

As you progress

- Gradually reduce the speed and size of the movements in all four directions, and try to keep them smooth.

- Repeat the entire exercise with your eyes closed.

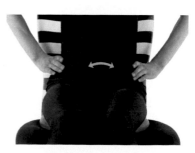

Hours on a clock face

Sit comfortably on a chair with or without a backrest.

Start from the centre position and tip your pelvis to 1 o'clock on an imaginary clock. Return to the centre. You need to move far enough to feel the movement without reaching your impairment.

Continue to move your pelvis to trace each hour on the clock face, ending at 12 o'clock, returning to the centre position each time. Notice your movements.

- Are they jerky?
- Do they follow a straight line?
- Are they equally spaced and accurate?

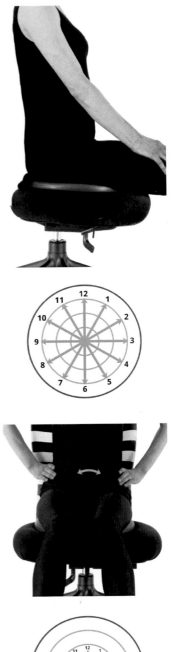

As you progress

- Reduce the size and speed of your movements.
- Try tracing the clock with your eyes closed.
- Try sitting *without* a cushion (or cushioned seat) and try this movement on different seats with different surfaces.

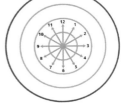

Letters of the alphabet

Sit comfortably on a chair with or without a backrest.

Move your pelvis to trace out the letters of the alphabet in upper or lower case, from A to Z. The centre of each letter should be located close to your centre position, and each letter can be drawn over the previous letter.

Aim to take at least 5 seconds to form each letter - this means you must "write" slowly. Keep going for a couple of minutes (you may not finish all of the letters).

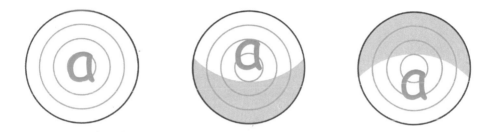

Train the movement close to the centre position without moving into your impairment.

As you progress

- Repeat these movements with your eyes closed, and focus on the moment-by-moment control of your fine movements.

- Trace out three or four different whole words – just slowly – for a couple of minutes.

- Choose new words so you can explore new movement paths.

- Trace out a series of numbers or invent your own special shapes to draw.

Flowing movements

Sit comfortably with relaxed lengthening of your whole spine, making sure your pelvis is also relaxed and free from restriction or discomfort.

Trace out a shape that allows a continuous flowing movement path such as a simple circle or letter "o", or a figure of "8" either upright or on its side. Repeat this movement and notice its flow, smoothness and accuracy. Watch out for any deviations from your intended movement path.

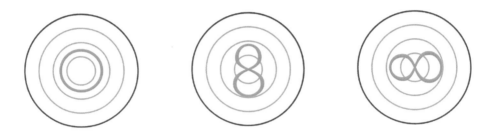

Adjust the speed, size and direction of movement to maximise fluidity and relaxation without discomfort.

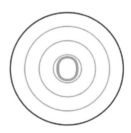

As you progress

- Try to reduce the muscle tension in all areas of your spine, from the top of your pelvis to the base of your head, and maintain relaxed breathing.

- Trace out new flowing movements, such as making a series of loops around each hour on a clock face (looping each time around the centre position).

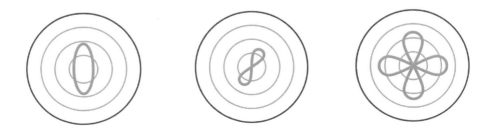

Mixing it up

It is important for your body to try out new and unusual movements to keep the challenge fresh for you and keep your attention focused. Think of it as drawing new movement pathways in your brain.

To this end, experiment with different ways of moving your spine close to the centre position. You can also:

- Revisit any of the exercises you have already tried.

- Try different positions – lying on your back with your knees bent, or on one side, all fours, or standing with your knees slightly bent.

- Change the angle of your hips or knees when you sit. If you sit on a chair that is higher than usual for you, your knees will be lower than your hips.

- Vary the speed of your movements, from fast or medium to slow.

- Vary the size of your movements – without losing control of the movement or your awareness of it. These might be movements extending to 50% on your movement map to tiny, almost imperceptible movements within 5% from the centre.

- Coordinate your movements with your breathing patterns.

- Notice which movements are smooth and which are jerky, and how they change when you do them at different speeds. Also notice which movements feel good – and do them more often!

- Remember that small, slow movements can usually be carried out without being noticed by other people, which means they can be done *anywhere*.

Working with your impairments

So far, the emphasis has been on having awareness of movements near and around the centre position, where your spine is the strongest and safer to load than anywhere else in its range of movement. Sitting in this way should result in less pain and stiffness. As long as you work within an area that is comfortable and *free of pain*, this should help your impairments to recede gradually.

For normal daily life, it is not possible to function by just remaining *near* the centre position; we sometimes need to use far more movement than that for activities such as getting dressed, gardening or playing sport.

For most longstanding conditions and more resistant impairments, you should also aim to restore and maintain your *flexibility*. This is where controlled, paced and "graded" stretches can help because they can also help to reduce impairments. However, these exercises should be individually tailored in order to improve flexibility and help restore functional mobility[56]. Make sure you have good, habitual control of movement around the centre position before starting a stretching routine. When improving your mobility, it is important to remember the spine is strongest near the centre position.

A basic paced stretch

- Lie down on a comfortable flat surface, to help you relax. Start with a slow, controlled movement in the direction of (but *short* of) your impairment and hold this position for 10 to 20 seconds. The next four examples show movements stretching forwards, but could also be for bending backwards or bending or rotating to one side.

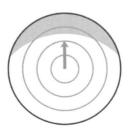

- Repeat the stretch three times in one session. Three times is usually the minimum number of repetitions, but this can usually be gradually increased, based on individual response.

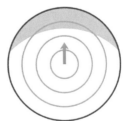

- Aim to fit in three to five sessions a day.

As you progress

- Over several days or weeks, extend the stretch further towards the edge of your impairment.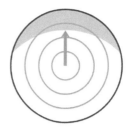

- As stretching becomes more familiar to you, gradually work further into the impairment. It may take many months to increase flexibility without increasing your symptoms.

- If the impairment is predictable and not changing, it is worth trying to nudge gradually into the impairment, as long as the discomfort settles within 20 minutes afterwards and your pain is not worse the day after.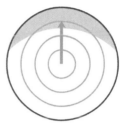

Your pain or discomfort should settle quickly after each stretching session. You will know if you are stretching too strongly or too far if you have a flare-up that lasts for more than 20 minutes. If this happens, try doing the stretches more gently next time.

You can also stretch in a direction that is *opposite* to your main impairment. This is often better tolerated, and you can stretch more firmly in this direction without causing the same level of discomfort, and with less risk of a delayed reaction. Stretching like this tends to: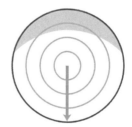

- Feel good at the time.
- Provide short-term relief.
- Can be repeated more often during the day.

A basic paced stretch is outlined here, but I recommend that you get advice on the best stretches for your specific condition.

13 Taking your focus away from your back

This is the final stage of learning to sit smartly – the level of "unconscious competence". Now your new movement skills are well established, and you are aware of your improved sitting habits. What's more, you notice when you revert to your old "habitual" positions. Sometimes you catch yourself sitting comfortably and with better posture without having planned to do so!

You are also able to move more easily and position your back more comfortably when you sit. The ideal, which you are fast approaching, is not to pay *too* much attention to your back.

People with lower back pain tend to think about their postures quite a lot,[63] but a constant focus on it can end up *increasing both* symptoms and muscle tension, making it harder to relax overall.

So the final stage of learning involves actively directing your attention *away* from your pelvis and lower back.

The best way to do this is to keep up with your breathing and relaxation routine. Both of these help to focus your attention away from your back area. Of course, from time to time you will need to re-focus on it for a while, at least, to carry out further testing, checking and training. This will help to maintain your level of competence and to reinforce your new sitting habits. It is like controlling a spotlight beam on a stage; it needs to be focused occasionally towards your back – just when it is needed – but the rest of the time, it attends to the main action.

This next chapter will help you to apply your new "smart" sitting skills to everyday situations in life.

14 Smart sitting in the real world

Having completed the training outlined in this book, you should be able to:

- Find your centre position.
- Relax and carry out movements while you are sitting down.

Some sitting positions will feel more comfortable than others, and you will find that some are better for you to feel movements in your back, to help relax your lower back, or to reduce the tension in your legs.

It is important to experiment with different sitting positions and to choose the most comfortable for your needs at any one time. You should be able to apply what you have learned to different sitting scenarios – on office chairs, hard dining-room chairs, upholstered car seats and soft couches – as well as to standing.

The aim is *always* to make sure you are capable of – and aware of – making relaxed, controlled movements, near the centre position. However, a poor chair will make that difficult.

The following pages highlight some of the important aspects of smart sitting that relate to common types of chairs found in everyday life. For added clarity, these examples are *exaggerations*.

With what you have learnt up to this point, you should be able to determine how much of each of these aspects you should utilise for best effect when sitting.

What is the ideal chair?

The ideal chair should provide comfortable support close to your spine's centre position, without preventing the movements you need to make. It should be capable of being adjusted so that it accommodates the needs of your body – rather than your body being forced into an undesirable or fixed position by the chair. These are the key points:

The surface of the seat

This should be soft enough to provide comfort and to encourage relaxation, but firm enough to provide sufficient support. This is always a case of trial and error. Fabric coverings are good because they provide "friction", which prevents unwanted sliding of your bottom. This is in contrast to the shiny, slippery surfaces like polished wood or smooth plastic.

The depth of the seat

This should fit your body very well, without the front edge of the seat pan digging into the back of your legs. Ideally, you should be able to tilt the seat pan both upwards and downwards.

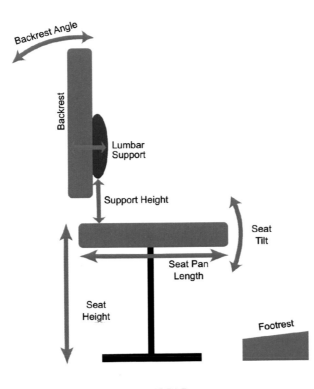

The height of the seat

This should be adjustable so that your head and arms are at a comfortable, relaxed and flexible working height. Your feet may need to be supported by a footrest to minimise pressure at the back of your thighs and knees. The same principle – of being able to function near the central position while promoting relaxed movement – applies to most joints and areas of the body, including the neck and arms, for low-intensity activities.

The backrest

This should provide comfortable support without restricting your movements. All the better if it is adjustable. Keeping your back in contact with the backrest will reduce your back pain.[67]

Lumbar supports

The size and position of the lumbar support should help to maintain the natural curves of the spine and allow the target segment to move near the centre position.

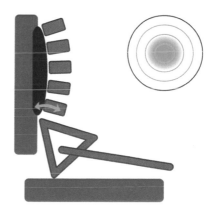

Whenever you sit, bear in mind the following:

- Keep your breathing relaxed and unrestricted.

- Hold minimal tension throughout the entire length of your spine.

- Stay aware of the centre position and try to move close to it – using the least amount of muscular effort possible.

- When you can easily identify and feel your centre position, adjust your chair to fit around it and allow for controlled, comfortable movement.

"Balanced" sitting in everyday chairs

Balanced sitting, as the name suggests, involves balancing your upper body, spine and pelvis on a chair in a way that promotes free, unconstrained, controlled movements of your spine and pelvis.

Having practised this previously, ideally on a wobble cushion or a soft upholstered or sprung seat, this kind of sitting is good to do on *any* chair and in *any* situation – whether at your desk, in a meeting, on a train or bus, or sitting in the doctor's waiting room. Musicians tend to sit like this, too. However, this kind of sitting differs from the training you have undertaken in terms of:

- How long you do it for. The mindful movement practice usually takes only a few minutes, but you may have to sit like this for longer in everyday situations. As a result, you may feel more tired to begin with.

- A tendency to remain still for longer periods of time compared with the larger movements often needed for movement training.

- A greater need for relaxed breathing and relaxed muscles when sitting for any length of time.

You can easily take advantage of this way of balanced sitting to continue your training.

Bear in mind that the seat may be backless, or it may have a backrest, in which case you should sit towards the front of the chair.

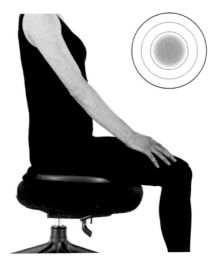

- Make occasional, small, slow, comfortable movements of your pelvis. If you do these slowly enough, they won't be noticed by anyone around you.

- Avoid holding any tension in your hips or legs.

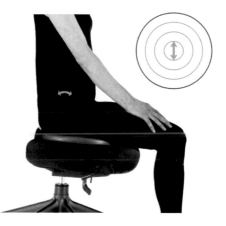

- Try to breathe from your diaphragm in a relaxed and unconstrained way, using just enough muscle tension to maintain an upright position, so that you feel the relaxed lengthening through the whole of your spine.

Now you know more about the movements you make, they do not *always* need to be mindful.

Using a lumbar support

You can use different types of lumbar supports to help maintain the shape of your lower back and keep it close to the centre position.

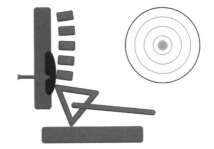

The type of support you choose should be *exactly* right for you and you only — that is, of the right size, in the right position, and with the right amount of padding. It should be firm enough to relieve your symptoms yet soft enough to allow you to move.

Large lumbar supports

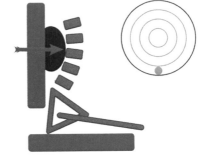

If the lumbar support is too big, your lower back may be pushed into excessive extension, which can lead to discomfort and increased tension in your back muscles.

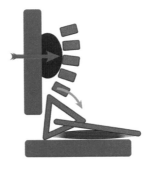

Your pelvis may roll too far forwards, so increasing extension of your lumbar spine, and this can increase tension in your back muscles. If your pelvis rolls forward too easily, it causes increased flexion of your hips, and increased tension in your hamstrings. It also tightens the sciatic nerves running down the back of your legs.

- Lumbar supports that are too big tend to slide you forwards on the seat, thus providing less effective support.

- A large support can be helpful for some flexion impairments when there are no leg or hip symptoms.

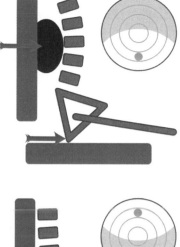

Small lumbar supports

If a lumbar support is too small, your pelvis may remain rotated backwards, and your lower back may remain in flexion.

A smaller lumbar support can be useful if you are trying to relax your back muscles, or if you have an extension impairment.

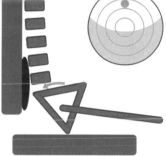

The position of the support

If the support is positioned too far up your back, the lowest part of your back may remain flexed and unsupported; the support will be ineffective for controlling the position of your pelvis.

Ideally you should place a small cushion or a lumbar roll at the top part of your pelvis or at the lower part of your back, to help roll the pelvis forwards and away from the fully flexed position. This lets you make a variety of movements, and allows your spine to make contact with both the lumbar support, and the back-rest, which helps reduce pain.[67]

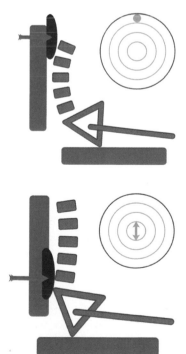

It may take some trial and error to find the best kind of lumbar support to suit your needs.

The angle of the seat-pan

Triangular wedges made out of foam are very useful, as is tilting the seat-pan downwards. Both of these allow your pelvis to roll forwards more easily towards the centre position. It is like sitting on a bar stool or a saddle chair, whereby your knees are lower than your hips, which reduces flexion in your hips and tension in your hamstrings, and takes the pressure off your sciatic nerves.

There is a problem with using wedges or using a down-tilting pan. That is, there is a tendency for your bottom to *slide forwards*. This means you may have to use counter-pressure through your feet and legs to hold your position. Furthermore, sliding forwards on a seat reduces the effectiveness of any backrest or lumbar support you use.

Tilting the seat-pan backwards (upwards)

This position tends to move you towards the *back* of the chair, so your pelvis and spine make firmer contact with the backrest and lumbar support. If you do tilt it upwards, make sure the front edge of the seat that comes into contact with the back of your legs (shown by the orange star) does not dig into the back of your legs or restrict the flow of blood.

This position of the seat pan works better when combined with a slightly reclined backrest.

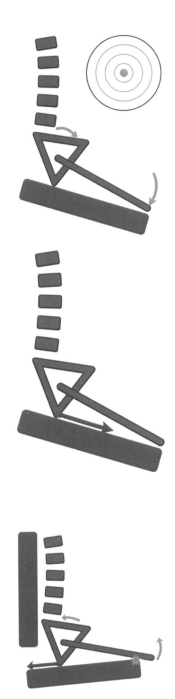

The angle of the adjustable backrest

What we consider to be the most comfortable kind of sitting is on a sofa, armchair or chair with an adjustable backrest. These seats demand less muscular effort than others, which is generally more relaxing. They also allows you to make more relaxed movements of your spine. The specific advantages are:

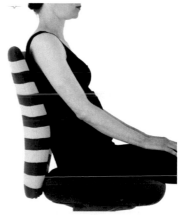

- Your spine is well supported simply because more of your upper spine is in contact with the backrest, thus the load is shared between your lower spine and your upper spine.

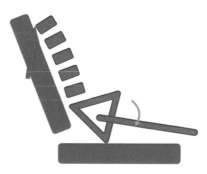

- The front of your hips are in an open position, which reduces flexion in the area.

- There is less tension in your hamstrings and less pressure on your sciatic nerves.

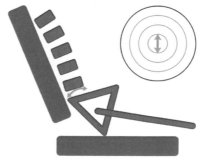

- Your can easily roll your pelvis forwards and backwards.

- The centre position can be reached with less effort.

However, if you recline too far back, there may be a tendency for:

- The upper part of your spine and neck to flex (in order to keep your head level).

- Your bottom to slide forward (making you use your feet and leg muscles to hold yourself in position).

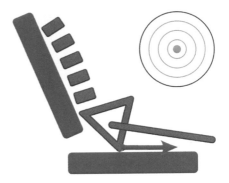

- Your pelvis and lower back to move away from the backrest, meaning there is less support for your lower back, which may move further into flexion.

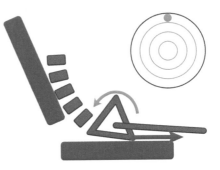

Sliding forwards on the seat-pan can be controlled by:

- Reclining the angle of the seat-pan (upwards at the knees).

- Using a footrest to keep your knees slightly higher than the level of your hips, so allowing some of the pressure to pass through your legs.

- Using a seat with good surface grip.

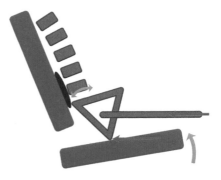

Car seats and driving

It is a good idea to check (when the car is stationary) whether you can move your pelvis a small amount so that you know you can make small movements; when it is safe to move. This can prevent or relieve your symptoms.

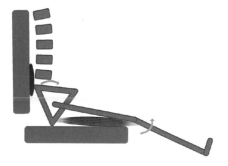

Sitting bolt upright, with the car seat pushed too far away from the foot pedals, is not usually the best position for driving. Not only does it tend to over-stretch the back of your legs, but it can also make it difficult to roll your pelvis forwards.

For a more comfortable sitting position while driving, you can try:

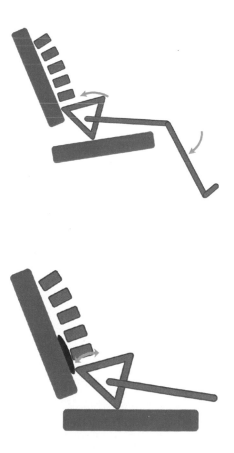

- Reclining the backrest to allow the pelvis to roll forwards more easily.

- Reclining the seat-pan to help limit forward sliding on the seat.

- Sliding the seat-pan forwards towards the wheel, so that your knees can bend a bit. This relaxes the back of the legs and reduces pressure on your hamstrings and sciatic nerves.

- Placing a small support behind your lower back, of a suitable size for you, to help your spine stay closer to the centre position. Remember, if you have an extension impairment, you will require less lumbar support.

Dealing with specific problems

Stiffness and muscle tension around your hips and pelvis can limit your ability to position yourself and move your lower back near the centre position. Here are some tips on how to minimise these problems.

Stiff hips

Stiffness in the hips can limit their ability to bend into flexion. Hip flexion is needed for the pelvis to rotate forward to achieve a good sitting position. This is common in conditions like osteoarthritis, rheumatoid arthritis, congenital conditions of the hip, and excessive tension in the posterior hip muscles. If you are affected you can try the following:

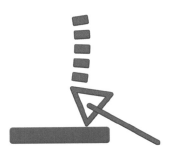

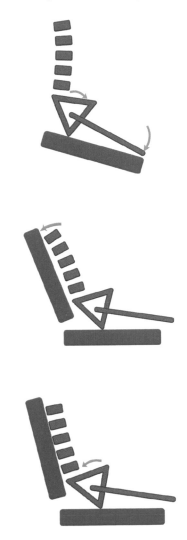

- Sit towards the front of a chair and lower your knees.

- Tilt the seat-pan forward, or sit on a foam wedge or a bar stool. When the knees are below the hips, it reduces the amount of flexion at the hips.

- Recline the backrest backwards, or position your knees below the level of your hips (or a combination of both).

- You can also reduce the size of any lumbar support you are using, which will reduce extension in your back and allow your pelvis to roll backwards.

Tense leg muscles

Muscle tension is often increased if you have back pain, usually in the back, the back of the hips, the hamstring area and the calf muscles. Irritation of the sciatic nerves can also increase tension in these muscles. Thus, back pain not only creates a localised problem; it also affects other areas, and your legs in particular, which has a knock-on effect on the way you sit.

Sitting with your pelvis rolled forward can increase the pressure on your sciatic nerves and make your hamstrings tense up. The tension is even greater if your knees are straightened out.

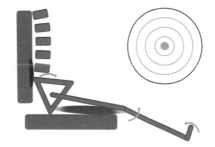

If your feet and toes are also pulled up (towards your head), your sciatic nerves will be affected even more.

To relieve tension in your legs:

- Recline the backrest.

- Allow your knees to bend more.

- Allow your feet to relax.

- Reduce hip flexion (as in hip stiffness page 94).

- Reduce the size of the lumbar support to reduce extension in your back.

- Relax and move your back close to the centre position.

- Choose a seat with a softer surface.

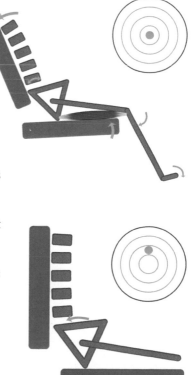

Movement impairments

Sometimes, an impairment can be large enough to prevent you from making comfortable movements near the centre position. Ignoring an impairment like this, in order to maintain a good centre position, will probably increase your symptoms. Therefore, you need to find an area that is *opposite* your area of impairment for making comfortable movements.

Large flexion impairments

Large flexion impairments may trigger symptoms when you try to adopt a good sitting position or when your functional movements cause you to move into areas of impairment. Good postural alignment with movement is not ideal when symptoms increase by trying to maintain that alignment.

You can help your spine into lumbar extension by using a larger lumbar support *without* forcing your back towards the extreme limit of extension. Make sure you are still able to move your pelvis and lower back.

When moving your back further into lumbar extension, it can be difficult to relax the muscles of your back. Changing your position and getting up and walking about may be necessary.

Any activities that involve more lumbar extension, such as walking or swimming, are more comfortable.

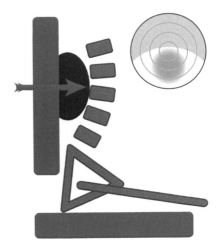

Large extension impairments

Large extension impairments tend to be uncomfortable when you try to adopt a good sitting position.

These types of impairment are usually more comfortable in positions that allow your back to bend slightly forward (into flexion).

Sitting with lumbar flexion, or slightly slumped, and using less lumbar support, should relieve your symptoms.

A reclining back-rest with minimal lumbar support can also help – just make sure that your lower back is not kept fully flexed and that you can still make movements.

When sitting in flexion with this type of impairment, increased muscle tension is usually not an issue.

Activities such as cycling and rowing, which involve more lumbar flexion, are more comfortable.

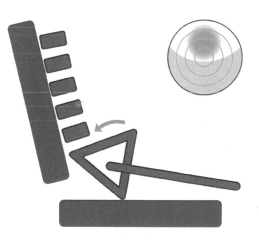

Closing comments

Mastering the skills in "smart sitting" takes time and careful, accurate practice, and you should continue to refine these skills until they are all second nature to you. They will continue to empower you with the knowledge and ability to take control of your body and spine when you are sitting down.

Your awareness of how to move and position your spine when sitting should be noticeably better than when you started the programme, and you now know how to move more comfortably, using less effort, and to move within your own area of movement impairment. Your habitual postures are easier to identify.

You are more aware that you are staying in one position, and of the position of your spine when you stay in that position. You have also developed an awareness of how much movement is available at your spine from your current sitting position.

Being empowered to move and find the best position for your own back allows you to adapt your seating environment to fit and suit your specific needs. In turn, having choices about your seating allows for more comfortable and relaxed movement so your spine does not remain "stuck" for long periods of time in any particular position.

Once you have mastered all of these skills, make sure you continue to practise controlling your focus of attention, taking it away from your spine for most of the time. You will be able to direct attention back to your spine as and when needed.

Remember that our bodies thrive on movement and exercise, so you should take frequent breaks from sitting whenever possible and avoid inactivity.

The key points are summarised on the next page.

Key points

I would like to leave you with a few key points for your continuing journey in smart sitting:

- Remember that sitting causes the pelvis to bend the lower back (into flexion) and thus reduces movement.
- You need to find your centre position.
- Minimise all muscle effort.
- Maintain relaxed breathing.
- Explore comfortable movements within your area of impairment.
- Check the accuracy of your movements using feedback.
- Focus your mind to feel movements on a moment-to-moment basis.
- Change the shape, speed and size of your movements.
- Exercise good control over your focus of attention.

From now on, you can enjoy *smart sitting* and moving more often.

References and further reading

1. Karayannis NV, Jull GA, Hodges PW. Physiotherapy movement based classification approaches to low back pain: comparison of subgroups through review and developer/expert survey. *BMC Musculoskelet Disord.* 2012 Feb 20;13(1):24. http://www.biomedcentral.com/1471-2474/13/24.

2. Ng SW, Popkin BM. Time use and physical activity: a shift away from movement across the globe: Declines in movement across the globe. *Obes Rev* 2012; 13(8):659–80.

3. Bauman A, Ainsworth BE, Sallis JF, Hagströmer M, Craig CL, Bull FC, *et al.* The descriptive epidemiology of sitting. *Am J Prevent Med* 2011; 41(2):228–35.

4. G. Shin G, D'Souza C, Liu YH. Creep and fatigue development in the lower back in static flexion. *Spine* 2009; 34(17):1873–78.

5. Lin CWC, McAuley JH, Macedo L, Barnett DC, Smeets RJ, Verbunt JA. Relationship between physical activity and disability in lower back pain: A systematic review and meta-analysis. *Pain* 2011; 152(3):607–13.

6. Van der Ploeg HP, Chey T, Korda RJ, Banks W, Bauman A. Sitting time and all-cause mortality risk in 222,497 Australian adults. *Arch Intern Med* 2012; 172(6):494–500.

7. Chau JY, Grunseit AC, Chey T, Stamatakis E, Brown WJ, Matthews CE, *et al.* Daily sitting time and all-cause mortality: a meta-analysis. *PLoS ONE* 2013; 8(11):e80000.

8. Van Daele U, Hagman F, Truijen S, Vorlat P, Van Gheluwe B, Vaes P. Differences in balance strategies between nonspecific chronic lower back pain patients and healthy control subjects during unstable sitting. *Spine* 2009; 34(11):1233–38.

9. Falla D, Gizzi L, Tschapek M, Erlenwein J, Petzke F. Reduced task-induced variations in the distribution of activity across back muscle regions in individuals with lower back pain. *Pain* 2014; 155(5):944–53.

10. Søndergaard KHE, Olesen CG, Søndergaard EK, de Zee M, Madeleine P. The variability and complexity of sitting postural control are associated with discomfort. *J Biomech.* 2010 Jul;43(10):1997–2001.

11. Hodges PW, Smeets RJ. Interaction between pain, movement, and physical activity: short-term benefits, long-term consequences, and targets for treatment. *Clin J Pain.* 2015 Feb;31(2):97–107.

12. Sung PS, Leininger PM. A kinematic and kinetic analysis of spinal region in subjects with and without recurrent low back pain during one leg standing. *Clin Biomech.* 2015 Aug;30(7):696–702.

13. Tsao H, Tucker KJ, Hodges PW. Changes in excitability of corticomotor inputs to the trunk muscles during experimentally-induced acute low back pain. *Neuroscience.* 2011 May 5;181:127–33.

14. O'Sullivan P. It's time for change with the management of non-specific chronic low back pain. *Br J Sports Med.* 2012 Mar 1;46(4):224–7.

15. Kiers H, van Dieën JH, Brumagne S, Vanhees L. Postural sway and integration of proprioceptive signals in subjects with LBP. *Hum Mov Sci.* 2015 Feb;39:109–20.

16. Silfies SP, Squillante D, Maurer P, Westcott S, Karduna AR. Trunk muscle recruitment patterns in specific chronic low back pain populations. *Clin Biomech.* 2005 Jun;20(5):465–73.

17. Sheeran L, Sparkes V, Caterson B, Busse-Morris M, van Deursen R. Spinal position sense and trunk muscle activity during sitting and standing in nonspecific chronic lower back pain: classification analysis. *Spine* 2012; 37(8):E486–95.

18. Claeys K, Brumagne S, Dankaerts W, Kiers H, Janssens L. Decreased variability in postural control strategies in young people with non-specific low back pain is associated with altered proprioceptive reweighting. *Eur J Appl Physiol.* 2010 Sep 8;111(1):115–23.

19. Nairn BC, Azar NR, Drake JDM. Transient pain developers show increased abdominal muscle activity during prolonged sitting. *J Electromyog Kinesiol* 2013; 23(6):1421–27.

20. Schinkel-Ivy A, Nairn BC, Drake JDM. Investigation of trunk muscle co-contraction and its association with lower back pain development during prolonged sitting. *J Electromyog Kinesiol* 2013; 23(4):778–786.

21. Hodges PW, Tucker K. Moving differently in pain: A new theory to explain the adaptation to pain. *Pain.* 2011 Mar;152(3):S90–8.

22. Yamato TO, Maher CG, Saragiotto BT, Hancock MJ, Ostelo RW, Cabral CM, *et al. Pilates for lower back pain.* Cochr Data Syst Rev, John Wiley & Sons 2015:1-71.

23. Pereira LM, Obara K, Dias JM, Menacho MO, Guariglia DA, Schiavoni D, *et al.* Comparing the Pilates method with no exercise or lumbar stabilization for pain and functionality in patients with chronic lower back pain: systematic review and meta-analysis. *Clin Rehabil* 2012; 26(1):10–20.

24. Liddle SD, Baxter GD, Gracey JH. Exercise and chronic low back pain: what works? *Pain.* 2004 Jan;107(1-2):176–90.

25. Akuthota V, Nadler SF. Core strengthening. *Arch Phys Med Rehabil.* 2004 Mar;85:86–92.

26. Mannion AF, Caporaso F, Pulkovski N, Sprott H. Spine stabilisation exercises in the treatment of chronic low back pain: a good clinical outcome is not associated with improved abdominal muscle function. *Eur Spine J.* 2012 Jan 24;21(7):1301–10.

27. Lederman E. The myth of core stability. *J Bodyw Mov Ther.* 2010; 14(1):84–98.

28. Scott SH. Optimal feedback control and the neural basis of volitional motor control. *Nat Rev Neurosci* 2004; 5(7):532–46.

29. Beevor CE. Croonian Lectures: Muscular movements and their representation in the central nervous system. Delivered before the Royal College of Physicians of London. *Br Med J* 1903; 2(2218):12-16.

30. Feldenkrais M. *Awareness Through Movement.* London: Arkana. 1990

31. Hillier S, Worley A. The effectiveness of the Feldenkrais method: a systematic review of the evidence. *Evid Based Complement Alternat Med* 2015; (Article ID 752160):1–12.

32. O'Sullivan K, McCarthy R, White A, O'Sullivan L, Dankaerts W. Can we reduce the effort of maintaining a neutral sitting posture? A pilot study. *Man Ther.* 2012 Dec;17(6):566–71.

33. Gilbert C. Better chemistry through breathing: the story of carbon dioxide and how it can go wrong. *Biofeedback.* 2005;33(3):100–4.

34. McLaughlin L, Goldsmith CH, Coleman K. Breathing evaluation and retraining as an adjunct to manual therapy. *Man Ther* 2011; 16(1):51–52.

35. Laffey JG, Kavanagh BP. Medical progress. *N Engl J Med* 2002; 347(1): 43-53.

36. Laird RA, Gilbert J, Kent P, Keating JL. Comparing lumbo-pelvic kinematics in people with and without back pain: a systematic review and meta-analysis. *BMC Musculoskelet Disord.* 2014;15(1):229:http://www.biomedcentral.com/1471-2474/15/229.

37. Tsao H, Danneels LA, Hodges PW. Issls prize winner: smudging the motor brain in young adults with recurrent lower back pain. *Spine* 2011; 36(21):1721–27.

38. Kuner R, Flor H. Structural plasticity and reorganisation in chronic pain. *Nat Rev Neurosci* 2016; 18(1):20–30.

39. Flor H, Braun C, Elbert T, Birbaumer N. Extensive reorganization of primary somatosensory cortex in chronic back pain patients. *Neurosci Lett* 1997;224(1):5–8.

40. Tsao H, Galea MP, Hodges PW. Driving plasticity in the motor cortex in recurrent low back pain. *Eur J Pain.* 2010 Sep;14(8):832–9.

41. Seminowicz DA, Wideman TH, Naso L, Hatami-Khoroushahi Z, Fallatah S, Ware MA, *et al.* Effective Treatment of Chronic Low Back Pain in Humans Reverses Abnormal Brain Anatomy and Function. *J Neurosci.* 2011 May 18;31(20):7540–50.

42. Schabrun SM, Elgueta-Cancino EL, Hodges PW. Smudging of the Motor Cortex Is Related to the Severity of Low Back Pain: *Spine.* 2017;Aug 1;42(15):1172-78.

43. O'Sullivan K, O'Keeffe M, O'Sullivan L, O'Sullivan P, Dankaerts W. Perceptions of sitting posture among members of the community, both with and without non-specific chronic low back pain. *Man Ther.* 2013 Dec;18(6):551–6.

44. Bowering KJ, Butler DS, Fulton IJ, Moseley GL. Motor imagery in people with a history of back pain, current back pain, both, or neither. *Clin J Pain* 2014;30(12):1070–75.

45. Sung W, Abraham M, Plastaras C, Silfies SP. Trunk motor control deficits in acute and subacute lower back pain are not associated with pain or fear of movement. *Spine J* 2015;15(8):1772–82.

46. Harris AJ. Cortical origin of pathological pain. *The Lancet* 1999;354(9188):1464–66.

47. Brumagne S, Janssens L, Knapen S, Claeys K, Suuden-Johanson E. Persons with recurrent lower back pain exhibit a rigid postural control strategy. *Eur Spine J* 2008;17(9):1177–84.

48. Verschueren S, O'Sullivan K, Van Hoof W, Dankaerts W. Lumbar proprioceptive deficits in sitting in patients with non-specific chronic lower back pain with a flexion pattern sub-classification. *Presented at the Joint World*

Congress of ISPGR and Gait and Mental Function. 2012;24-28 June:Trondheim, Norway.

49. Sato K, Kikuchi S, Yonezawa T. In vivo intradiscal pressure measurement in healthy individuals and in patients with ongoing back problems. *Spine* 1999;24(23):2468-74.

50. Suni J, Rinne M, Natri A, Statistisian MP, Parkkari J, Alaranta H. Control of the lumbar neutral zone decreases lower back pain and improves self-evaluated work ability: A 12-month randomized controlled study. *Spine* 2006; 31(18):E611–20.

51. O'Sullivan K, O'Dea P, Dankaerts W, O'Sullivan P, Clifford A, O'Sullivan L. Neutral lumbar spine sitting posture in pain-free subjects. *Man Ther* 2010;15(6):557–61.

52. Little P, Lewith G, Webley F, Evans M, Beattie A, Middleton K, *et al.* Randomised controlled trial of Alexander technique lessons, exercise, massage (ATEAM) for chronic and recurrent back pain. *BMJ* 2008;337(2):a884.

53. Wang H, Weiss KJ, Haggerty MC, Heath JE. The effect of active sitting on trunk motion. *J Sport Health Sci* 2014; 3(4):333–37.

54. Grossman P. Defining mindfulness by how poorly I think I pay attention during everyday awareness and other intractable problems for psychology's (re)invention of mindfulness: Comment on Brown K W, West A M, Loverich T M, & Biegel G M. 2011. *Psychol Assess* 2011;23(4):1034–40.

55. Gard T, Holzel BK, Sack AT, Hempel H, Lazar SW, Vaitl D, *et al.* Pain attenuation through mindfulness is associated with decreased cognitive control and increased sensory processing in the brain. *Cereb Cortex* 2012;22(11):2692–2702.

56. Nijs J, Meeus M, Cagnie B, Roussel NA, Dolphens M, Van Oosterwijck J, *et al.* A modern neuroscience approach to chronic spinal pain: combining pain neuroscience education with cognition-targeted motor control training. *Phys Ther* 2014;94(5):730-8.

57. Bushnell MC, Čeko M, Low LA. Cognitive and emotional control of pain and its disruption in chronic pain. *Nat Rev Neurosci* 2013;14(7):502–11.

58. Nijs J, Kosek E, Van Oosterwijck J, Meeus M. Dysfunctional endogenous analgesia during exercise in patients with chronic pain: to exercise or not to exercise? *Pain Physician* 2012;15(3S):ES205–13.

59. O'Keefe M. How to move on from back pain. *Irish Independent* 2016 Aug 29;12 h&l.

60. Rogers KH. Luton R, Biggs H, Biggs R, Blignaut S, Choles A G, Palmer C G, and Tangwe P. Fostering complexity thinking in action research for change in social-ecological systems. *Ecol Soc* 2013;18(2):Art 31.

61. George PJ, ManipPhysio M, Smith AJ, Goucke R, Moseley GL. Seeing it helps: movement-related back pain is reduced by visualization of the back during movement. *Clin J Pain* 2012;28(7):602–8.

62. Claus AP, Hides JA, Moseley GL, Hodges PW. Thoracic and lumbar posture behaviour in sitting tasks and standing: Progressing the biomechanics from observations to measurements. *Appl Ergon.* 2016 Mar;53:161–8.

63. O'Sullivan K, Verschueren S, Van Hoof W, Ertanir F, Martens L, Dankaerts W. Lumbar repositioning error in sitting: Healthy controls versus people with sitting-related non-specific chronic lower back pain (flexion pattern). *Man Ther* 2013;18(6):526–32.

64. Willigenburg NW, Kingma I, van Dieën JH. Center of pressure trajectories, trunk kinematics and trunk muscle activation during unstable sitting in lower back pain patients. *Gait Post* 2013;38(4):625–30.

65. Claus AP, Hides JA, Moseley GL, Hodges PW. Is "ideal" sitting posture real? Measurement of spinal curves in four sitting postures. *Man Ther* 2009;14(4):404–08.

66. Van Diest I, Verstappen K, Aubert AE, Widjaja D, Vansteenwegen D, Vlemincx E. Inhalation/exhalation ratio modulates the effect of slow breathing on heart rate variability and relaxation. *Appl Psychophysiol Biofeedback* 2014 Dec;39(3-4):171–80.

67. Vergara M, Page A. Relationship between comfort and back posture and mobility in sitting-posture. *Appl Ergon* 2002;33(1):1–8.

Index

A

all fours (position) 44–45, 71
anxiety 9
awareness of position 9, 11, 17, 34

B

back pain
  caution 3
  delayed reactions 12, 79
  injury 21
  muscle tension 8
  position awareness 9, 10
  reduced mobility 8
  stabilisation 8
balanced sitting 86
brain reorganisation 10
brain training 12, 69, 77
breathing
  hypocapnia 9
  need to practise 65
  relaxation 67, 68
  when lying 40, 67
  when sitting 41, 68
  when standing 47

C

caution / medical advice 3
centre position 42, 65, 85
chairs
  backrest 85, 91
  depth of seat 84
  driving 93
  height of seat 85
  lumbar support 85, 88, 89
  seat-pan 90
  surface of seat 84
  the ideal chair 84
checking yourself. *see also* testing yourself
  feedback 55–58, 60, 66
  pelvic movements 56
closing your eyes 38, 63
combined impairments 25

comfort 3, 42, 51, 65
competence (learning) 33–34

D

driving 93

E

exercise
  duration/repetition 12, 66
  progression 69
  symptom-free 26, 69
extension 15
extension impairments 24, 97
external feedback 55, 57–60
eyes (closed) 38, 63

F

feedback
  external 55, 57–60
  internal 55, 60–63, 69
flexion 14
flexion impairments 24, 26, 96
focus of attention 34, 77, 81

H

habits
  brain training 3, 11, 65
  habitual sitting 10, 28, 49, 81
hips (stiff) 94
hypocapnia 9

I

ideal chair 84
ideal posture 35, 36
illness (serious) 3
impairments / problems
  combined 25
  extension 24, 97
  flexion 24, 26, 96
  functional impact 26
  lateral 25
  mapping 17, 51–52

multi-directional 25, 26
    stretching 78
incompetence (learning) 33
injury to back 21
internal feedback 55, 60–63

L

lateral impairments 25
learning (stages of)
    checking yourself 55
    conscious competence 34, 65
    conscious incompetence 33, 55, 65
    unconscious competence 34, 81
    unconscious incompetence 33, 37
leg muscle tension 88, 93, 95
lengthening of spine 35, 39, 47, 65
lumbar supports
    large 88
    position of 89
    small 89
lying (position) 40, 42–43, 58, 67, 70

M

medical caution 3
mindful movement
    active exploration 11, 69
    description 11
    internal feedback 55
    need to practise 8, 55
    visualisation 69
mindfulness 11, 69
mobility (reduced) 8, 24
mortality rates 7
movement maps
    creation of 20–25
    explanation / role 17, 20
    orientation 18, 19
    range of movement 18
    visualisation 17, 20, 62
movements. see also pelvic movements
    extension 15
    flexion 14
    size (smaller) 69, 72, 74
    speed (slower) 69, 72, 74
moving without pain 3
muscle contractions 8

muscle tension
    affect on movement 38
    breathing 9
    legs 93, 95
    lengthening 35, 39, 47, 65
    role of 9
    when sitting 29, 30, 39, 81

N

neurological deficits 3
neutral spine 10

P

pain 8, 69
pain-free movements
    delayed pain 12, 79
    need to practise 12, 66
    stabilisation of 8
    symptom free 26, 66, 69
pelvic movements
    clock face 74
    compass points 73
    flowing movements 76
    letters of alphabet 75
    right parts to move 56
    size of 42
    speed of 38
    when lying 42, 70
    when on all fours 44, 71
    when sitting 46, 72–77
pelvic position
    centre position 10, 47
    extension 15, 61
    flexion 14, 61
pilates 8
position awareness 9, 10, 17, 34
posture (ideal) 35
    sitting 36
    standing 35
problems. see also impairments; muscle
        tension
Problem sitting 27–29
proprioception 9

R

range of movement 18, 51–52

relaxation
  breathing 40–41, 67–68, 81
  lengthening 39–40, 47

S

seats. see chairs
segment (target) 13–15
serious illness 3
sitting
  balanced 86
  ergonomic 7
  examples of 83–97
  flexion limit 27
  ideal posture 36
  impairments 26, 53–54, 96–97
  mortality 7
  poor control 8
  rigid and upright 29
  staying at the limit 28
  the ideal chair 84
sitting bones 13
spine
  anatomy 13
  extension 15
  flexion 14
  lenthening 17, 39, 47, 65
  target segment 13, 17
standing (ideal posture) 35
stretching 69, 78
symptoms
  moving without 12, 26, 66, 69
  prediction of 24

T

target segment 13, 17
tension in muscles
  breathing 9
  effect of 8, 38
  focus of attention 81
  leg muscles 93, 95
  lengthening 35, 39, 47, 65
  when sitting 29–30, 39
testing yourself. *see also* checking
      yourself
  breathing when sitting 41
  centre position 47

  habitual 49
  impairments 51–54
  when lying 42–43
  when on all fours 44–45
  when sitting 46, 49, 53
therapists 60
training (retraining)
  brain 11
  breathing 67, 68
  clock face 74
  compass points 73
  flowing movements 76
  focus of attention 81
  letters of alphabet 75
  progression 69
  when lying 67, 70
  when on all fours 71
  when sitting 68, 72–76

V

visualisation 17, 20, 60–63

W

walking (with flexion impairment) 26
wobble cushions 46, 66

Blank movement maps for you

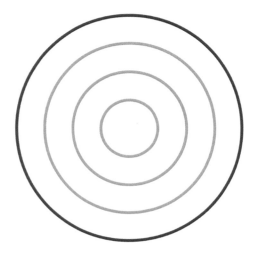

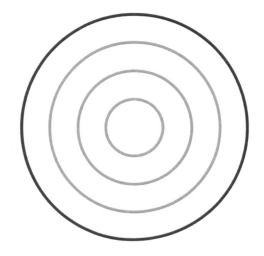